"I highly recommend this informative book. In it you [...]
evidence that will help inform your health-related decis[...]

from the foreword by **Dónal O'Mathúna**, PhD, a[...]
University College of Nursing; and associate professor, School of
Nursing & Human Sciences, Dublin City University, Ireland

"I strongly recommend Dr. Larimore's new book as a much-needed and intensely evidence-based resource on natural medicines. . . . Anyone reading this book will gain the skills needed to ask and answer the right questions about whether to and how to incorporate natural medicines as part of their healthy lifestyle."

Reid B. Blackwelder, MD, FAAFP, professor and chair, Department of
Family Medicine, Quillen College of Medicine; past president,
American Academy of Family Physicians

"Dr. Larimore undertakes a heroic effort to assemble and synthesize a vast amount of data on commonly used natural medicines. The result is an entirely digestible and ultimately useful guide for patients and practitioners alike."

Matthew A. Ciorba, MD, gastroenterologist,
Washington University, St. Louis, MO

"A terrific handbook that sheds light on an exceedingly opaque topic. In the world of brain health, navigating the landscape of herbs, vitamins, and supplements can be particularly complex and treacherous. Dr. Larimore's approach is direct and comprehensive and will certainly help numerous patients and their families make informed and safe decisions."

Jacob N. Hall, MD, clinical assistant professor of neurology and neurological
sciences, Stanford Center for Memory Disorders, Palo Alto, CA

"Dr. Larimore presents a truly practical approach in his *Natural Medicine Handbook*. The book defines wellness- and disease-related natural medication advice while also emphasizing the importance of a healthy lifestyle. This book provides extensive information and data that can be easily translated into excellent advice for patients."

Sandra L. Argenio, MD, past president, Florida Academy of Family Physicians;
Family Medicine Emeritus Faculty, Mayo Clinic Florida, Jacksonville, FL

"An outstanding compendium outlining the clinical data associated with a large number of supplements. Dr. Larimore, as a physician who has been involved in the natural medicine marketplace for decades, brings a scientific and objective perspective to the field, carefully showing us what we know and don't know about each supplement."

Matthew Budoff, MD, professor of medicine, UCLA; Endowed Chair of
Preventive Cardiology, Lundquist Institute, Torrance, CA

"The world of natural medicines is a jungle of misinformation and confusion. Dr. Larimore has dissected that confusion to provide reliable, independent information that will help you find the safest path forward to discern what is truly safe and effective."

Robert Griffith, MD, FAAD, Alabama Dermatology Associates, Northport, AL

"Walt Larimore helps us understand that diet, exercise, and moderate habits are the foundations for our health, and he also empowers us to use nonprescription remedies without a doctor's order when they are safe and effective. . . . If you are open to the best available information for a healthy lifestyle, this handbook can help you. If you want the best information about nonprescription remedies for the minor problems that affect us all, this handbook can help you. If you, your family, and your friends are confused by clever marketers who take your money for fake products or even for reliable pills that simply don't work, this handbook can help you."

Marc Raphaelson, MD, FAAN, FAASM, neurologist, Veterans Administration Medical Center, Martinsburg, WV

"This well-researched natural medicine handbook is informative and practical. It ranks the natural products with potential benefits and harm—and everything in between. The material is presented in such a way that one can research by the supplement one is considering or by accessing the medical condition a person is addressing. What a wonderful resource for all of us."

Mary Anne Nelson, MD, FAAFP, family physician, Cedar Rapids, IA

"This book takes the guesswork out of natural supplements. Dr Larimore does a great job laying out the positives and the negatives of natural medicines."

Steve Foley, MD, FACOG, Regenerative Health and Wellness, Colorado Springs, CO

"Due to all the hype and sheer volume of advertisements, internet searches, and word-of-mouth recommendations touting the 'amazing' benefits of any number of vitamins, supplements, and natural remedies, not a day goes by without my being asked about at least one of these topics. Thank you, Dr. Larimore, for creating this much-needed resource, which so clearly lays out what has been backed up by sound studies, what has been shown to have little or no positive effect on a particular medical condition, and what is frankly dangerous to patients. You have made my life a bit easier and my medical advice to patients inquiring about such supplements much better informed!"

Susan Henriksen, MD, family physician, Glen Rock, PA

"As a busy family physician, I am always searching for high-yield information that is easy to read and provides meaningful value to my practice and my patients. This latest book by Dr. Larimore hits all of those marks and gives me the confidence I need to practice holistic evidence-based medicine."

Huy Luu, DO, DABFM, International Medical Center, Almaty, Kazakhstan

"In our current age of overwhelming information regarding our health, Dr. Larimore's book cuts through the chaos. He uses scientific evidence paired with his expertise as a medical doctor to make this a comprehensive and reliable guide. Highly recommended!"

Cherec Morrison, MD, family physician, Tulsa, OK

"I would recommend this well-researched, concise book to all my patients, especially in an age when more and more people are seeking out and using natural medicines."

Sam Kammerzell, DO, family physician, Tulsa, OK

The
NATURAL
MEDICINE
HANDBOOK

Foreword by **Dónal O'Mathúna, PhD**
author of *Alternative Medicine: The Options, the Claims, the Evidence, How to Choose Wisely*

The
NATURAL
MEDICINE
HANDBOOK

The Truth about the Most Effective Herbs, Vitamins, and Supplements for Common Conditions

Walt Larimore, MD

In consultation with the experts at
ConsumerLab.com and ***Natural Medicines*™**

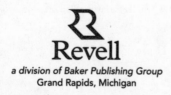

Revell

a division of Baker Publishing Group
Grand Rapids, Michigan

© 2021 by Walter L. Larimore, MD

Published by Revell
a division of Baker Publishing Group
PO Box 6287, Grand Rapids, MI 49516-6287
www.revellbooks.com

Printed in the United States of America

Library of Congress Cataloging-in-Publication Data
Names: Larimore, Walter L., author.
Title: The natural medicine handbook : the truth about the most effective herbs, vitamins, and
    supplements for common conditions / Walter L. Larimore, MD.
Description: Grand Rapids, Michigan : Revell, a division of Baker Publishing Group, 2021. |
    Includes index.
Identifiers: LCCN 2020038867 | ISBN 9780800738211 (paperback) | ISBN 9780800740368
    (casebound)
Subjects: LCSH: Alternative medicine—Handbooks, manuals, etc.
Classification: LCC R733 .L367 2021 | DDC 610—dc23
LC record available at https://lccn.loc.gov/2020038867

The proprietor is represented by WordServe Literary Group, www.word serveliterary.com.

21 22 23 24 25 26 27   7 6 5 4 3 2 1

In keeping with biblical principles of creation stewardship, Baker Publishing Group advocates the responsible use of our natural resources. As a member of the Green Press Initiative, our company uses recycled paper when possible. The text paper of this book is composed in part of post-consumer waste.

To Amanda, Tod, and Meredith
along with the writers and staff at
ConsumerLab.com and *Natural Medicines*™

Contents

Contents

Foreword

The market for herbal remedies, dietary supplements, and natural medicines continues to grow. For decades now, the interest in these products has not decreased. But neither have the concerns that Dr. Walt Larimore and I have been writing about for twenty years. Foremost among these is the myth that because something is "natural," it must be safe. The natural world contains many poisonous and dangerous things. Just because something is "natural" or has "natural" on the label does not make it safe; it also doesn't mean it will do you any good.

We should all ask the following questions before taking *any* remedy or treatment: What's the evidence that this works? If it works, will it work for my condition? What sorts of side effects might it have? Was it manufactured to the highest possible standards? Was it tested to make sure that what's on the label is in the bottle? And does it contain anything it shouldn't have in it?

The challenge when we are looking at a natural medicine, whether in a store aisle or while surfing the internet, is that we may not know where to find answers to these questions. Even if we do, they may be buried in a professional publication or a hard-to-understand reference.

But now you have in your hands a really helpful, evidence-based guide. Dr. Larimore is to be commended for investigating the current evidence on many commonly used supplements and remedies and providing clear summaries along with helpful charts and tables. He has combined forces with two excellent sources of reliable evidence: ConsumerLab.com and *Natural Medicines*™. These professional organizations continuously monitor the evidence being produced about natural remedies. Dr. Larimore then weaves this evidence, and that of other reports, into highly readable overviews of what we currently know about natural remedies for common conditions.

I highly recommend this informative book. We all know to look before we leap. You should look in here before you grab your next natural remedy. You may not like everything you read because it might not confirm what you thought, heard, or hoped was the case. But you will find reliable, independent evidence that will help inform your health-related decisions.

Dónal O'Mathúna, PhD, associate professor, Helene Fuld Health Trust National Institute for Evidence-Based Practice in Nursing and Healthcare, College of Nursing, Ohio State University, Columbus, Ohio; Executive Committee, Cochrane US Network, and former director, Cochrane Ireland

Abbreviations

A1C	glycated or glycosylated hemoglobin, hemoglobin A1C, or HbA1C
AACC	American Association for Clinical Chemistry
AAD	American Academy of Dermatology
AAN	American Academy of Neurology
AARP	American Association of Retired Persons
ACC	American College of Cardiology
ACG	American College of Gastroenterology
ACS	American Cancer Society
ACSM	American College of Sports Medicine
AD	Alzheimer's disease
ADA	American Diabetes Association
AGA	American Gastroenterological Association
AHA	American Heart Association
AHAs	alpha hydroxy acids
AIDS	acquired immune deficiency syndrome
ALA	alpha-lipoic acid
AMA	American Medical Association
AND	Academy of Nutrition and Dietetics
ASCVD	atherosclerotic cardiovascular disease
ASDS	American Society for Dermatologic Surgery
ASU	avocado soy unsaponifiables
BHB	beta-hydroxybutyrate
BMI	body mass index
BP	blood pressure
BSS	bismuth subsalicylate
CAG	Canadian Association of Gastroenterology
CAGR	compound annual growth rate
CAM	complementary and alternative medicine
CBD	cannabidiol

CDC	Centers for Disease Control and Prevention
CFU	colony forming unit
CLA	conjugated linoleic acid
CoQ10	coenzyme Q10
CRAP	chronic recurrent abdominal pain
CRN	Council for Responsible Nutrition
CVD	cardiovascular disease
DASH	Dietary Approaches to Stop Hypertension
DHA	docosahexaenoic acid
DHEA	dehydroepiandrosterone
DMAA	1,3-dimethylamylamine
DMAE	dimethylaminoethanol or deanol
DO	Doctor of Osteopathic Medicine
DrPH	Doctor of Public Health
DSHEA	Dietary Supplement Health and Education Act of 1994
EDTA	ethylenediamine tetraacetic acid
EPA	eicosapentaenoic acid
EU	European Union
FAAFP	Fellow of the American Academy of Family Physicians
FDA	Food and Drug Administration
FODMAP	fermentable oligo-, di-, mono-saccharides, and polyols
FOS	fructo-oligosaccharides
FTC	Federal Trade Commission
GCBH	Global Council on Brain Health
GERD	gastroesophageal reflux disease
GI	gastrointestinal
GLA	gamma-linolenic acid
GMP	good manufacturing practices
GNC	General Nutrition Centers
GOED	Global Organization for EPA and DHA
GOS	galacto-oligosaccharides
H2	histamine 2 receptor
HBP	high blood pressure
HCA	hydroxycitric acid
HDL	high-density lipoprotein, healthy cholesterol, good cholesterol
Hg	mercury
HHS	Health and Human Services
HIV	human immunodeficiency virus
HMB	hydroxymethylbutyrate
HMG-CoA	3-hydroxy-3-methyl-glutaryl-CoA reductase or HMGR
HTN	hypertension
IBD	inflammatory bowel disease
IBS	irritable bowel syndrome
IBS-C	irritable bowel syndrome with constipation
IBS-D	irritable bowel syndrome with diarrhea

14

IBS-M	irritable bowel syndrome with alternating (mixed) constipation/diarrhea
IDSA	Infectious Diseases Society of America
IU	international units
JAMA	*Journal of the American Medical Association*
LAC	L-acetylcarnitine or acetyl-L-carnitine
LDL	low-density lipoprotein, lethal cholesterol, or bad cholesterol
mcg	micrograms
MCI	mild cognitive impairment
MD	Medical Doctor
mg	milligram
mg/dl	milligrams per deciliter
MIND	Mediterranean-DASH Diet Intervention for Neurodegenerative Delay
MLM	multi-level marketing
mm	millimeter
MPH	Master of Public Health
NACB	National Academy of Clinical Biochemistry
NAG	N-acetyl glucosamine
NCCAM	National Center for Complementary and Alternative Medicine
NCCIH	National Center for Complementary and Integrative Health
NDMA	N-nitrosodimethylamine
NIA	National Institute on Aging
NIH	National Institutes of Health
NMBER	*Natural Medicines* Brand Evidence-based Rating
NSF	National Sanitation Foundation
OSA	obstructive sleep apnea
OTC	over-the-counter
oz	ounce
PCB	polychlorinated biphenyls
PCOS	polycystic ovarian syndrome
PEA	palmitoylethanolamide
PharmD	Doctor of Pharmacy
PhD	Doctor of Philosophy
PPI	proton pump inhibitor
ppm	parts per million
PQQ	pyrroloquinoline quinone
PSO	pumpkin seed oil
PTH	parathyroid hormone
PUFA	polyunsaturated fatty acid
RD	registered dietitian
RDN	Registered Dietitian Nutritionist
R/S	religion and spirituality
RVD	rotavirus diarrhea
SPF	sun protection factor
SSRI	selective serotonin reuptake inhibitor

TD	travelers' diarrhea
TG	triglycerides
THC	tetrahydrocannabinol
TSH	thyroid stimulating hormone
UC	ulcerative colitis
UK	United Kingdom
UL	upper tolerable intake level
URTI	upper respiratory tract infection
US	United States
USD	US dollars
USDA	United States Department of Agriculture
USP	United States Pharmacopeia
USPSTF	US Preventive Services Task Force
UTI	urinary tract infection
UV	ultraviolet
UVA	ultraviolet A
UVB	ultraviolet B
WHO	World Health Organization
WW	Weight Watchers

Disclaimer

This book contains advice and information relating to health and medicine. It is designed to help you become a more informed consumer of medical and health services. It is not intended to be exhaustive and should not be considered a substitute for medical or other advice from your healthcare professionals. You are advised to consult your healthcare professionals in regard to matters relating to your health and, in particular, regarding matters that may require diagnosis or medical attention.

I've worked overtime to ensure the accuracy and evidence-based nature of the information contained within this book as of late 2020. The endorsers, reviewers, consultants, author, and publisher expressly disclaim responsibility for any adverse effects resulting from the application of the information contained herein.

In most of the chapters, I discuss specific products and manufacturers based on the recommendations or reports of multiple independent testing labs and trustworthy sources. You need to know the following:

1. I have no financial ties to *any* of these organizations and products.
2. Although I have endorsed ConsumerLab.com and *Natural Medicines*™ for over twenty years, I have never received financial remuneration from either. ConsumerLab provides me with complimentary access to their website, and *Natural Medicines* and *Prescriber's Letter*™ also allow me, as one of their peer-review experts, to utilize their web materials.

3. All cost information shared with you on specific products derives from the best information available in late 2020 when the book was being completed and are in US dollars (USD). Of course, prices on products frequently change over time and can vary at different stores or websites. Consider any cost information herein to be general information only.

In the various summary charts in most of the chapters, the recommendations are based primarily on the Safety and Effectiveness Ratings contained in *Natural Medicines*. These ratings assume you are using high-quality, uncontaminated products in typical doses and are otherwise a healthy individual. Supplements that are safe for healthy individuals might not be safe for patients with certain conditions. In other words, most natural medicines (herbs, vitamins, or supplements) are never appropriate for some patients due to concomitant disease states, potential drug or food interactions, or myriad potential clinical factors. I highly recommend that you involve your family physician or personal pharmacist before utilizing *any* natural medicine, especially if you are taking prescription medications or have any medical or psychological illnesses.

The website addresses recommended and cited are offered as a resource. They are not intended in any way to be or imply an endorsement on the part of the author, the reviewers, the endorsers, the consultants, or the publisher (Baker Publishing Group). Also, we cannot vouch for their content or availability for the lifetime of this book. For most website references, I've used tinyURLs, which will "not break in email postings and never expire."[1] By entering the tinyURL symbols (e.g., tinyURL.com/ABCDE) into your internet browser, the reference, if still available online, should appear.

Introduction

Natural medicines (herbs, vitamins, and supplements) are trendy across most of the developed world. According to a 2019 report,[1] the global natural medicines market was valued at about 140 billion USD in 2018 and could reach over 216 billion USD by the year 2026, at a compound annual growth rate (CAGR) of 5.5 percent. The report indicates, "Asia-Pacific is expected to be the largest market for dietary supplements in 2026, accounting for a significant share of the global market, followed by North America and Europe. However, the market in Europe and North America will continue to be very profitable due to the lack of price pressure, which is common in the Asia-Pacific region."[2] Even more optimistic research estimated that the global dietary supplements market is expected to reach over 220 billion USD in 2022 while growing at a CAGR of 8.8 percent.[3]

The amount of information regarding options for almost every problem known is overwhelming, and unfortunately, as I'll show you, much of it is inaccurate. Nevertheless, for the conditions covered in this book, I'll provide you with evidence-based recommendations from the most recent and reliable medical studies.

Because no one person could be an expert in all of the topics I'll address, I'll quote dozens of trusted natural medicine specialists from around the globe. I've enlisted the assistance of respected healthcare professionals (listed in the acknowledgments) to review this book to help ensure that the information it contains is accurate, evidence-based, objective, and medically reliable. I will tell you not only what is safe and effective but even more importantly what is potentially unsafe or ineffective—as well as what therapies have no or insufficient reliable evidence one way or the other.

As I detail in the appendix, I've evaluated aproximately 1300 natural medicines and interventions for about 550 conditions or indications. You may be quite shocked to learn how few can actually be recommended. Two-thirds of the extensively advertised and commonly sold substances I've reviewed for this book don't have evidence of safety or effectiveness. They would not only be a waste of time and money but in some cases could also be dangerous.

I'll also reveal to you the often hard-to-find information about the least expensive natural medications that are safe and effective for these common conditions.

It's important to note that the recommendations in this book are only for adults who are not pregnant or breastfeeding. Many natural medicines

Of the ~1,300 natural medicines and interventions I evaluated for ~550 conditions/indications

★★★★★	83	6%	150	11%
★★★★	67	5%		
★★★	88	7%	260	22%
★★	69	5%		
★	103	10%		
⊗	888	67%	888	67%

KEY

★★★★★	I recommend considering in almost all cases (Effective & Likely Safe)
★★★★	I recommend in many to most cases (Likely Effective & Likely Safe)
★★★	I recommend in some cases (Effective & Possibly Safe)
★★	I recommend in a few cases (Likely Effective & Possibly Safe OR Possibly Effective & Possibly Safe)
★	I recommend in unusual cases (Possibly Effective & Possibly Safe)
⊗	I recommend against using (Insufficient Evidence, Possibly Ineffective, Possibly Unsafe, Ineffective, or Unsafe)

have different safety and effectiveness ratings for pregnant women, breast-feeding women, and children.

I'm extremely grateful for the invaluable assistance of the experts in natural medicines from two organizations, ConsumerLab.com and *Natural Medicines*™, which provided me with access to their vast internet resources. In addition, each chapter, each recommendation, and each warning that I give you has been reviewed by these experts.

I want to provide you with the most up-to-date, accurate information that will allow you to not only find safe, effective, and economical options to consider but also avoid potentially dangerous, unproven, and money-wasting natural medicines.

I could not practice medicine the way I do (nor even begin to think about writing a book like this) without the practical materials these two organizations make available, by subscription, to me, my patients, and you, my readers.

ConsumerLab.com

ConsumerLab.com, LLC, is a leading provider of independent test results and information to help consumers and healthcare professionals identify the best-quality health and nutrition products. It publishes results of its tests in comprehensive reports at a subscription website, www.Consumer Lab.com, along with expert answers to many common questions about natural medicines. They frequently post news reports and information about recalls and warnings. ConsumerLab conducts an annual "Survey of Vitamin & Supplement Users," and its research is cited regularly by the media, in books, and at professional meetings.

ConsumerLab claims to have "perhaps the highest testing standards of any third-party group certifying the quality of dietary supplements" and to be "the only third-party verification group that freely publishes its testing methods and quality criteria/standards." Their standard is to test products, whenever possible, for each of the following:

- Identity: Does the product meet recognized standards of identifying all ingredients and the level of quality claimed on the label?

- Strength: Does the product contain the amount of each ingredient claimed on the label?
- Purity: Is the product free of specified contaminants?
- Disintegration: If a tablet, does it break apart correctly so that it may be absorbed?

Products that pass all four of the tests are approved and are eligible to bear the ConsumerLab "Approved Quality Product Seal" on their labels, which guarantees to consumers that the specific product carrying the seal has met ConsumerLab's standards and has passed all of ConsumerLab's tests for ingredient quality. The seal also indicates the specific ingredients of the product laboratory-tested by experts. In addition to the merchandise it selects to review, ConsumerLab enables companies of all sizes to have the quality of their products tested for potential inclusion in its list of approved products.

I especially like that ConsumerLab also gives the typical cost (in USD) of each product they review, which helps consumers compare the price of products. It's an invaluable resource to help readers determine which products contain what they need at the best value. To this end, they also provide their "Top Picks" for each natural medicine tested.

For example, ConsumerLab updated its review of vitamin C products in July 2020. All twenty-one tested products were "Approved." This is quite an improvement from their 2017 tests, which revealed problems with 20 percent of vitamin C supplements (none of the failing products were included in the current review). ConsumerLab chose three products as their "Top Picks" in the categories of pill, gummy, and powder.

The cost to obtain 500 mg of vitamin C from each product they tested, based on the price they paid, ranged from one cent to $2.80. However, among these products, the suggested daily doses ranged from 63 mg to 5,000 mg. With so broad a range, it's clear that you can't just follow instructions from a label; therefore, you have to choose a product that will provide the amount of vitamin C you actually need. ConsumerLab's "Top Picks" will help you do that. Their reviews also list vegan, gluten-free, and kosher products.

Since its founding in 1999, ConsumerLab has tested more than 5,600 products, representing over 850 different brands, and nearly every type of popular supplement for adults, children, and pets. Subscribers to ConsumerLab also have access to the online *Natural and Alternative Treatments™ Encyclopedia*.

Natural Medicines™

Natural Medicines, formerly known as the *Natural Medicines Comprehensive Database*, is also a subscription website and provides authoritative, independent information and resources on natural medicines as well as complementary, alternative, and integrative therapies. They provide health professionals and the public with interactive tools and over 1,250 monographs on the safety, effectiveness, and cautions for food, vitamins, herbs, and supplements and an additional 150 monographs on health and wellness topics. For each condition or diagnosis, *Natural Medicines* advises about each substance or therapy with two ratings:

1. SAFETY: "Likely Safe," "Possibly Safe," "Insufficient Evidence for Safety," "Possibly Unsafe," "Likely Unsafe," or "Unsafe." Meredith Worthington, PhD, former director and senior editor at *Natural Medicines*, writes, "Our 'Likely Safe' rating means that an ingredient has good evidence of safe use and would generally be considered appropriate to recommend."
2. EFFECTIVENESS: "Effective," "Likely Effective," "Possibly Effective," "Insufficient Evidence for Effectiveness," "Possibly Ineffective," "Likely Ineffective," or "Ineffective."

These ratings are explained in detail in chapter 4. One caution from *Natural Medicines* about the "Possibly Effective" rating: "A product might be rated 'Possibly Effective' for one condition but be rated 'Likely Ineffective' for another condition, depending on the evidence." Furthermore, by "Possibly Effective," they mean "this product has some clinical evidence supporting its use for a specific indication; however, the evidence is limited by quantity, quality, or contradictory findings. Products rated 'Possibly Effective' might be beneficial, but do not have enough high-quality evidence to recommend for most people."

Natural Medicines also has extensive information on health and wellness topics (i.e., everything from "Acupressure" to "Zero Balancing"), including many complementary and alternative medicine therapies. I also love their industry-leading NMBER® (*Natural Medicines* Brand Evidence-based Rating) for over 185,000 commercial brand products. NMBER provides an objective, scientific rating for most commercially available natural medicines and rates each from 1 to 10, with 10 being the highest. I do not recommend any product unless it's rated 8 out of 10 or higher by NMBER. *Natural Medicines* licenses its content to WebMD®, so much of what you read on WebMD about natural medicines comes from *Natural Medicines*.

I'm delighted that these two organizations granted me permission to use and adapt some of their wide-ranging content. Both organizations make most of their information available via subscription, and I think each subscription is worth its weight in gold. Group subscriptions are available to organizations such as faith communities, community groups, and social clubs. Also, many public libraries have (or upon request will purchase) a subscription that will allow you access to them.

However, please note that the ConsumerLab and *Natural Medicines* reviews are continually updated; therefore, you should strongly consider subscribing (or having access) to one or both if you want the latest information on these topics or products and if you want their other content (i.e., latest recalls and warnings, answers to common questions, interactions with tests or other medications, etc.). For example, in April 2020 I turned in the manuscript for this book. When I reviewed it again in October 2020, I had to make numerous updates. By the publication date of April 2021, there will likely be even more. So you'll need to keep up with any new information on conditions you may have or supplements you are either taking or considering.

To that end, ConsumerLab is offering readers of this book a free twenty-four-hour pass to review three major ConsumerLab.com product reviews mentioned in the book: Multivitamins & Multiminerals, CoQ10, and Fish Oil. You can access them at www.ConsumerLab.com/DrWalt. Also, *Natural Medicines* is offering a discount on the consumer editions of their online resources. Visit www.naturalmedicines.com and use promo code LARIMORE10 at checkout to receive a 10 percent discount on a subscription to *Natural Medicines*.

PART ONE

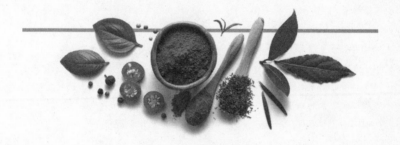

1

Natural Medicines Are Popular

It was an embarrassing night! I was hosting the first of what would turn out to be 854 episodes of the prime-time cable TV show *Ask the Family Doctor*. The show ran for five years, starting on America's Health Network, which two years later became Fox's Health Network. I had never done television before but was fortunate to be chosen from scores of far-more-experienced TV doctors to be one of the hosts for this live nightly national television show.

Before our inaugural broadcast on March 25, 1995, each of the show hosts had received extensive training. There were sixteen of us: the eight primary hosts, like me, worked Monday through Friday. We each had a live two-hour program, and the first hour of each broadcast was rerun during the overnight hours. We each had a substitute to cover the Saturday and Sunday shows. Based on this training and our practice experience, we were each prepared to answer questions about common maladies as well as interview experts on a wide variety of topics of interest to our viewers. However, I was *not* prepared for the first questions that night:

1. Does vitamin C work for colds?
2. What multivitamin should I take?
3. What supplement can I use for brain health and memory?

Three strikes. I didn't have a clue on any of these questions. But we had been trained to explain that if we didn't know the answer to an inquiry, we would promise to research it and answer the inquiry on the next edition of the program.

What I quickly learned those first few weeks of my program was that

- the public had an insatiable interest in natural medicines and alternative medicine,
- I knew very little about either,
- I needed a crash course in the truth, whatever it was, about complementary and alternative medicine (CAM), and
- the term *natural medicines* included herbal products, vitamins, and dietary supplements.

My expertise grew by leaps and bounds as I attended conferences and participated in distance learning with scores of experts. This allowed me to begin incorporating evidence-based information about natural medicines and CAM into my patient care, speaking, writing, and radio and TV programs.

My growing expertise led to two bestselling books that I coauthored with Dónal O'Mathúna, PhD: *Alternative Medicine: The Christian Handbook* (2001), which was updated and revised to *Alternative Medicine: The Options, the Claims, the Evidence, How to Choose Wisely* (2008). Both books did very well because the use of natural medications was hugely popular. It still is.

Billions Are Spent

Natural medicines are an approximately $30 billion industry in the US, with over 100,000 products on the market in 2018.[1] In 2020, *Natural Medicines*™ listed over 185,000 products.[2]

A 2019 consumer survey by the Council for Responsible Nutrition (CRN) announced, "Dietary supplement use reaches an all-time high." CRN added that "the use of dietary supplements among US adults increased ten percent over the past decade," and "77 percent of US adults take dietary supplements, as opposed to just 65 percent in 2009." The CRN survey revealed, "Among all the age groups, adults between the ages 35–54 have the highest usage of dietary supplements at 81 percent." It was 79 percent for US adults ages 55 or older and a striking 70 percent for those ages eighteen to thirty-four.[3]

Additionally, CRN found, "While vitamin/mineral supplements remain the most popular category among supplement users, the overall use of herbals/botanicals has significantly increased in the past five years. In 2019, 41 percent of supplement users reported they had taken herbals/botanicals in the past twelve months—up 13 percentage points from 2013."[4]

Another 2019 national survey reported 86 percent of Americans take natural medicines, especially vitamins and dietary supplements[5]—with 48 percent of adults taking vitamins and 39 percent taking supplements—most to "maintain health and prevent disease."[6] While yet another national survey showed that 52 percent of US adults reported the use of two natural medications a day[7] while 10 percent reported using at least four such products daily.[8] Although these percentages vary from source to source, depending upon who and how they surveyed, the point is that natural medicines are *very* popular.

What are the top reasons people take supplements? It varies by age group, but some themes run across the generations:[9]

18–34 years	35–54 years	55+ years
Overall Wellness (42%)	Overall Wellness (47%)	Overall Wellness (49%)
Energy (37%)	Energy (33%)	Fill Nutrient Gaps (33%)
Hair, Skin, Nails (28%)	Fill Nutrient Gaps (32%)	Bone Health (31%)
Immune Health (25%)	Immune Health (31%)	Heart Health (29%)
Fill Nutrient Gaps (22%)	Hair, Skin, Nails (23%)	Healthy Aging (28%)
Weight Management (21%)	Digestive Health (21%)	Joint Health (23%)

What are the most popular natural medicines for adults? In its "2020 Survey of Supplement Users," ConsumerLab.com reported:

Despite a slight decrease, vitamin D (-0.4 pts) remained the most popular supplement, purchased by 66 percent of respondents. With its continued rise in popularity, magnesium secured its place as the second most popular supplement and is used by 53.5 percent of respondents, surpassing [third place] fish oil. CoQ10 remained in fourth place this year, followed by multivitamins (42.4 percent, -1.3 pts), probiotics (38.9 percent, -2.7 pts), curcumin and turmeric (34.8 percent, -9.9 pts), vitamin C (including rose hips, 34.5 percent, -1.0 pt), B-complexes (31.2 percent, -1.1 pts), and vitamin B12 (cobalamin, 30.3 percent, +2.2 pts). Among the top 50 supplements, 30 declined in popularity, while only 19 showed an increase.

CRN reported that among the US adults they surveyed, multivitamins were the most popular dietary supplement (58 percent) followed by vitamin D (31 percent), vitamin C (28 percent), protein (21 percent), calcium and vitamin B or B complex (20 percent each), and omega-3 fatty acids/fish oil (16 percent).[10]

Again, the disparate results reflect different populations surveyed and different survey tools. For example, ConsumerLab surveyed 9,782 US adult subscribers (with over 82 percent taking at least four different supplements daily). In contrast, the CRN survey included a US sample of 2,006 adults, of whom only 1,529 considered themselves supplement users.[11]

Natural medicines are not only popular with adults; their use is also relatively common among children and adolescents. A 2020 CDC study reported that 34 percent took at least one while 7 percent took two or more of them. Most often-used were multivitamin-mineral products by almost 24 percent.[12]

People Believe Natural Medicines Are Healthy and Safe

The National Center for Complementary and Integrative Health (NCCIH) writes, "A lot of people believe that when it comes to medicine, 'natural' is better, healthier, and safer than 'unnatural' or synthetic drugs." They add, "Some people also believe that 'natural' products are safe because they believe these medicines are free of chemicals."[13] Around the world, people seem sold on the marketing claims that these products will allow them to avoid the "toxic, unnatural drugs" foisted on them by "the evils of Big Pharma" that "seeks enormous profits over the health and well-being of the humans it serves."[14]

An article in *Science-Based Medicine* adds, "Supplements are marketed as safe, natural, and effective, and there is no question that messaging has been effective."[15] CRN proclaims, "Consumer confidence in products and trust in industry remain strong. The majority of US adults—87 percent—have overall confidence in the safety, quality, and effectiveness of dietary supplements. . . . Additionally, . . . 78 percent of Americans perceive the dietary supplement industry as being trustworthy."[16]

The Bottom Line: Potential Dangers

It appears consumers of all ages in the Asia-Pacific, North American, and European regions have come to believe natural medicines are risk-free magic bullets for health and wellness as well as for treating every common malady.

Globally, people are in love with natural medicines and often use them across all age groups and for a wide variety of reasons. The popularity and use of these products have been increasing every year for decades, and most believe they are both safe and effective.

Unfortunately, false advertising and inflated claims are the norm. In addition, in the US contaminated and potentially dangerous products are not rare. Shockingly, these hazards are being withheld from consumers. In the next chapter, I share the truth and reveal the secrets that some natural medicine marketers are hoping you won't ever learn.

2

Natural Medicines Are Problematic

I find most of my patients are surprised to learn that, as JoAnn Manson, MD, chief of the division of preventive medicine at Brigham and Women's Hospital in Boston, writes, "Most supplements on the market [in the US] are not tested for either efficacy or safety."[1] *Natural Medicines*™ explains, "Most dietary supplements cannot claim to treat, cure, or prevent a disease. Doing so makes them legally unapproved drugs."

Unfortunately, the Food and Drug Administration (FDA) and the Federal Trade Commission (FTC) often must issue warning letters to companies whose "advertisements and labels tout the supplements' ability to treat or cure Alzheimer's, cancer, and myriad other diseases. The warning letters specifically call out the manufacturers for making unapproved drug claims and deceptive statements."[2] *Natural Medicines* explains that "many supplement companies bank on the ignorance of consumers and continue to skate this line. It can sway those with serious medical conditions away from using proven therapies."

"Even food products that are allowed to make specific health claims have not been 'approved' by the FDA the way that drugs are," says Dr. Meredith Worthington. "These health claims indicate that the FDA 'acknowledges' that the food product(s) may have evidence of benefit, but this process is not the same as the approval process for drugs."

A 2018 editorial in the *Journal of the American Medical Association* (*JAMA*) reported, "Clinicians and patients should be aware that the US FDA is not authorized to review dietary supplements for safety and efficacy prior to marketing."[3] This is unfortunate because, like *any* medication, *natural* medications have the potential to cause harm. I often say, "If a substance has *no* side effects, then you can be 100 percent sure it has *no* effects."

Besides the fact that "makers of dietary supplements are not required to prove effectiveness, safety, or quality of a product before marketing their products," even more disturbing is that manufacturers of natural medicines "are not required to report [the] discovery of adverse effects to the FDA."[4]

Quality and Safety Concerns

Quality and safety concerns are not new. In testimony before the US Congress in 2010, Tod Cooperman, MD, president and founder of ConsumerLab .com, said, "Based on tests of over 2,000 dietary supplements representing over 300 different brands, we find that one out of four has a quality problem. Problems have been found in products from every size of manufacturer and are most common in herbal supplements, multivitamins, and products with ingredients that are newer to the market."

Cooperman added, "Our most recent tests of herbal supplements show that 46 percent contained less than their expected amounts of key compounds." Of course, the problem with this is that if you don't get enough of the natural medicine you might need, it's not likely to work, and you've just wasted your money. Imagine buying an antibiotic, an anti-seizure drug, or a heart drug that you thought contained a particular amount of medicine, but it did not. You'd be justifiably outraged!

But that's not the only problem with these products. ConsumerLab cites the following common troubles with natural medicines sold in America:

- Tablets that won't break apart properly to release all of their ingredients and therefore are much less likely to be absorbed.

- A lack of proper labeling because they had too few or too many nutrients.
- Deceptive labeling suggesting more ingredients than provided or components that are not in the product at all.
- Products that contain potentially dangerous, even cancer-causing or heavy metal, contaminants.
- A lack of voluntary warnings that could help consumers avoid potential problems, such as ingredients in amounts above known tolerable levels, and a lack of public access to adverse event reports filed by manufacturers with the FDA.
- Faulty products left on the market due to inaction by manufacturers or "quiet" recalls announced to retailers but not to the public.
- The illegal addition of prescription, experimental, or unapproved drugs, particularly those sold for "erectile dysfunction," "bodybuilding," "brain health," and "weight loss."

In 2010, based on ConsumerLab tests, if you purchased a natural medicine in the US, you had between a one-in-two and a one-in-four chance of buying a product that did not meet even minimum standards for safety. You'd assume this would have been fixed by now, but you'd be wrong. In early 2020, ConsumerLab reported that about one in five supplements in the US and Canada that they tested did not meet one or more quality parameters. This is true even though ConsumerLab's testing tends to focus on the more popular and established brands that would be expected to have the *best* findings.

ConsumerLab also reported in early 2020 based on information from the FDA that 51 percent of 598 US dietary supplement manufacturing facilities audited from October 1, 2018, through September 30, 2019, failed inspections and received letters of noncompliance with good manufacturing practices (GMP). ConsumerLab received the results under the Freedom of Information Act.

The good news is that the high-water mark in the failed inspections in US facilities was 70 percent in 2012. "Although an improvement over past years," says Cooperman, "the most recent FDA audits show that, overall, dietary supplement manufacturers need to do a lot better." He added,

"Consumers often express concern about supplement ingredients from China, but the US is doing no better than China based on this limited sampling. People may also be surprised that four out of five facilities were noncompliant in Germany, where many herbal supplements have drug status. However, our tests have shown issues with some products from Germany."

The FDA noted a median of four infractions at facilities that received notices but did not release a list of the specific violations of each facility. Nevertheless, the most common breaches, each observed at more than 15 percent of noncompliant facilities, included the following:

- not establishing product specifications for the identity, purity, strength, or composition of the finished dietary supplement (25.25 percent)
- not establishing or following written procedures for quality control operations (21.64 percent)
- not producing batch records, which include the complete information relating to the production and control of each batch (15.08 percent)

If you don't think the situation is bad enough, this may make the hair on the back of your neck stand up: a 2015 study by the New York attorney general concluded, "DNA testing . . . shows that, overall, just twenty-one percent of the test results from store-brand herbal supplements verified DNA from the plants listed on the products' labels—with 79 percent coming up empty for DNA related to the labeled content or verifying contamination with other plant material."[5] In other words, they found that if you purchase one of the tested herbal supplements, you had a four-in-five chance of being duped.

In February 2019, FDA Commissioner Dr. Scott Gottlieb said, "The growth in the number of adulterated and misbranded products—including those spiked with drug ingredients not declared on their labels, misleading claims, and other risks—creates new potential dangers."[6]

Science writer Markham Heid reported, "Despite recent studies that find supplements are frequently contaminated or that the best way to get nutrients is through food, Americans' interest in supplements is only growing. And experts say many supplement users don't recognize or appreciate the risks that accompany the use of these products."[7] In 2018, a study in *JAMA* reported, "From 2007 through 2016, 776 adulterated dietary supplements were identified by the FDA, and 146 different dietary supplement companies were implicated."[8]

A perfect recent example surrounds the growing popularity of cannabidiol or CBD. The market size is soaring at about 35 percent CAGR and could reach 1.3 billion USD by 2024.[9] The *New York Times* reports, "We are bombarded by a dizzying variety of CBD-infused products: beers, gummies, chocolates and marshmallows; lotions to rub on aching joints; oils to swallow; vaginal suppositories for 'soothing,' in one company's words, 'the area that needs it most.'"

Even CVS and Walgreens have "announced plans to sell CBD products in certain states."[10] The *Times* adds, "Many of these products are vague about what exactly CBD can do. . . . Yet promises abound on the Internet, where numerous articles and testimonials suggest that CBD can effectively treat not just epilepsy but also anxiety, pain, sleeplessness, Crohn's disease, arthritis, and even anger."[11] The FDA sent out a flurry of letters warning companies not to make medical claims.[12]

In 2015, the FDA reported it found that many CBD-labeled products contained very little CBD.[13] Two years later, another study published in *JAMA* found that in eighty-four CBD products sold online, forty-three (51 percent) had more CBD than advertised, and twenty-six (31 percent) had less. Also, eighteen of the eighty-four products (21 percent) contained THC (the psychoactive component of marijuana), with none listed on the label.[14]

By 2020, things had not improved. Another study analyzed CBD products purchased over the counter and reported, "Of the 25 products, only three were within ±20% of label claim. Fifteen were well below the stated claim for CBD; two exceed claims in excess of 50%; and 5 made no claims. . . . THC content for three products exceeded the 0.3% legal limit [and]four products—primarily marketed for vaping—were adulterated with synthetic cannabinoids." The authors concluded, "It appears that most product label claims do not accurately reflect actual CBD content and are fraudulent in that regard." For the consumer, products that exceed legal THC levels may jeopardize their employment status (i.e., a failed drug test), and those adulterated with synthetic cannabinoids can result in serious adverse health effects.[15]

Regulatory Concerns

I bet you're finding these facts almost unbelievable. "After all," you might argue, "people around the world respect the FDA for its pharmaceutical policies. No other country is as rigorous in protecting the public. We can rely on our prescriptions and over-the-counter medications to be high-quality, safe, and effective." And you are 100 percent correct.

Unfortunately, the same is *not* true for natural medicines. Dr. Manson compares "the current regulatory environment to 'the Wild West.'"[16] How did this ever come to be? Scott Gavura, writing for *Science-Based Medicine*, explains, "It's a consequence of legislation deliberately designed to weaken the FDA's ability to regulate and provide oversight of supplements. The Dietary Supplement Health and Education Act of 1994 (DSHEA) was an amendment to the US Federal Food, Drug, and Cosmetic Act that established the American regulatory framework for dietary supplements. It effectively excludes manufacturers of these products from many of the requirements that are in place for prescription and over-the-counter drugs. Amazingly, it puts the requirement to demonstrate harm on the FDA rather than the onus on the manufacturer to show a product is safe and effective."[17]

Natural Medicines adds, "One of the biggest differences between drug regulations and dietary supplement regulations is the approval process. There is no approval process for dietary supplements. As long as supplements contain dietary ingredients that were either already used in supplements before DSHEA (1994), or established as reasonably safe since then, they can be sold to consumers lawfully. . . . This is very different from drugs, which must go through an extensive approval process before entering the market. Basically, drugs are assumed unsafe until proven safe, whereas supplements are assumed safe until proven otherwise."

Adverse Reaction and Effectiveness Concerns

Besides the many regulatory difficulties with natural medications, there are many other potential dangers consumers may not be aware of. For example, "Although many people don't realize it, dietary supplements can cause serious health concerns when taken incorrectly. They are a common reason for calls to US Poison Control Centers, and dietary-supplement-related calls are on the rise," says a report from *Natural Medicines*.

In 2017, researchers published data showing that in just over ten years, "US Poison Control Centers received nearly 275,000 calls related to dietary supplements."[18] That's one call every twenty-four minutes! *Natural Medicines* writes, "The majority of the calls involved miscellaneous dietary supplements, followed by botanicals and hormonal products. Of these, seventy percent related to dietary supplement use in children younger than six years old. These exposures were mostly accidental, so it's important to store dietary supplements out of the reach of children."

Another critical issue is the possibility of the interactions and direct toxicities of natural medicines. The NCCIH warns, "Although there is a widespread public perception that herbs and botanical products in dietary supplements are safe, research has demonstrated that these products carry the same dangers as other pharmacologically active compounds. Interactions may occur between prescription drugs, over-the-counter drugs, dietary supplements, and even small molecules in food—making it a daunting challenge to identify all interactions that are of clinical concern."[19]

Now, I'm not a guy that's for big government and lots of regulations. But in healthcare, I think they are often necessary and helpful. And in the case of natural medicines, one could have predicted that the DSHEA's weakening of the rules protecting consumers would increase the risks of manufacturers taking shortcuts, which could result in inconsistent product quality and even irresponsible behavior from some manufacturers. Unfortunately, that's precisely what we find when we look at supplement sales today.

Worse yet, it has led to far too many catastrophic harms suffered by consumers. In 2019, researchers from Harvard T.H. Chan School of Public Health found that of the single-supplement-related adverse event reports in children and young adults, "approximately 40 percent involved severe medical outcomes, including death and hospitalization. Supplements sold for weight loss, muscle building, and energy were associated with almost three times the risk for severe medical outcomes compared to vitamins. Supplements sold for sexual function and colon cleanse were associated with approximately two times the risk for severe medical outcomes compared to vitamins."[20]

There's also the issue of effectiveness. Despite ubiquitous advertising to the contrary, for natural medicines as a broad category, there is very little reliable evidence to support most of the claims. "With a few exceptions," Gavura writes, "the research done on dietary supplements is unconvincing and largely negative."[21] The National Institute on Aging (NIA) adds, "Some ads for dietary supplements in magazines, online, or on TV seem to promise that these supplements will make you feel better, keep you from getting sick, or even help you live longer. Often, there is little, if any, good scientific research supporting these claims. Supplements may cost a lot, could be harmful, or simply might not be helpful."[22]

Is There Any Hope for Consumers?

By now, you may be thinking that I'm against natural medicines. Nothing could be further from the truth! I've recommended and promoted them for over two decades; however, I use the same standards for my natural medication recommendations as I do for my pharmaceutical and over-the-counter medication recommendations: I only prescribe or suggest products that are both safe *and* effective.

I have yet to find a patient or a consumer who doesn't want *all* of their medicines—prescription, over-the-counter, *or* natural—to be manufactured to the highest quality standards and to have accurate labeling. I think we all could agree that the product label should accurately describe what's in the bottle, and there should be no exceptions to this. And yes, there should be no substituted ingredients and absolutely no contaminants at all. Again, no exceptions.

One attorney very familiar with false-advertising cases against supplement manufacturers wrote that there is a "long history of expensive and time-consuming litigation over dietary supplements, much of which could be avoided if Congress ditched DSHEA and passed a law regulating dietary supplements and their marketing meant to protect consumers, not the industry. Here's another prediction: that's not going to happen."[23]

However, a false advertising case against a manufacturer of a supplement for brain health that was settled in 2020 (see chapter 6, Brain Health—Part 1) "could be one of the largest consumer class settlements in the country . . .

awarding tens of millions in damages."[24] As a result, shady manufacturers "are keeping a close eye on the U.S. Food and Drug Administration (FDA) as it rolls out a plan to overhaul protocols for controlling and monitoring dietary goods," wrote one law firm. "FDA Commissioner Dr. Scott Gottlieb said the overhaul will be the most significant of its kind in the 25 years since the Dietary Supplement Health and Education Act (DSHEA) was passed."

But until Congress repeals or revises DSHEA or the FDA completes its promised revision, the only hope for the average health professional, patient, or consumer considering a natural medication is to ask the questions I've adapted from PBS's 2016 *Frontline* special, "Supplements and Safety."[25]

1. *Has the product triggered any health warnings or sanctions?* Searching the FDA's website for a list of all recalls (tinyurl.com /y5kxnwbu) will identify if the product in question has problems. ConsumerLab notifies its subscribers of significant warnings and recalls. Nevertheless, given the few resources put into monitoring supplement safety issues, a lack of notices is no assurance of quality or safety.

2. *Is the product too good to be true?* While supplement makers cannot legally make unfounded claims of efficacy, it's not hard to find these claims on products or on the internet. Again, it's important to note that there are no magic bullets out there. Outlandish claims should not be believed.

3. *Is there evidence that the supplement does what it promises?* Look to reputable sources that summarize the evidence without bias. If there's no good evidence supporting any efficacy claims, it's a giant red flag that the product is probably bogus. As I've mentioned, my favorite nonbiased source for whether a natural medicine is safe and effective is *Natural Medicines*.

Frontline recommends you do a little research before taking any natural medicine. I would wholeheartedly agree. However, I must warn you that, in general, the internet is an unreliable place to do your research. One study reported that among health websites, retail websites presenting information on products they were selling had the lowest level of medical accuracy (only 9 percent). On the other hand, government websites (.gov) and websites of national organizations (.org) had the highest level of accuracy (81 and 73 percent, respectively). Note, however, that even these "reputable" sources weren't close to 100 percent accurate! Shockingly, the same study reported that educational websites (.edu sites, ebooks, peer-reviewed articles) only had 50 percent accurate medical information. The majority of the books found by search engines either provided outdated or irrelevant information. Blogs and websites of individuals are even worse, having low rates of accuracy (26 and 30 percent, respectively).[26]

However, there are several trustworthy, medically accurate, unbiased, and evidence-based sources of information I highly recommend:

- The National Institutes of Health (NIH) has summaries about the most commonly consumed supplements—vitamins and minerals—in a series of fact sheets.[27]
- The US National Library of Medicine's MedlinePlus has similar information about drugs, herbs, and supplements.[28] For a deeper dive into the science behind a specific supplement, explore the Library of Medicine's PubMed Dietary Supplement Subset.[29]
- Resources are also available for specific groups. For example, the Department of Defense offers information about the safety of specific supplements for service members.[30] Older adults can find resources specifically designed for them by the FDA,[31] FTC,[32] and NIA.[33]
- The NIH includes the National Center for Complementary and Integrative Health (NCCIH), which provides information about complementary health products and practices—including many natural medicines.[34]

These sites can give you general information on natural medicines but are of very little help when it comes to choosing specific products. Therefore, *Frontline*'s number one recommendation, and mine also, is that before you purchase *any* vitamin, herb, or supplement, you ask this question: *Has the product been tested by an independent lab that makes the data available to the public?* This is critical and is the only real protection health professionals and consumers have from unscrupulous manufacturers, untrained salespeople, and fraudulent, contaminated, or dangerous products. The independent quality testing labs (such as ConsumerLab.com, the National Sanitation Foundation [NSF® International], Labdoor, and the United States Pharmacopeia [USP®]) purchase these products from the same places you and I would (big-box stores, health food stores, pharmacies, the internet, etc.) and test them or have them tested for quality.

As I mentioned earlier, my two go-to organizations for evidence-based information on natural medicines as well as which specific products to recommend are ConsumerLab.com and *Natural Medicines*™. ConsumerLab uses a variety of labs for its tests to "Approve" particular products, while *Natural Medicines* highlights products that are USP®-"Verified." They may also, in the future, include other certifications in their commercial product database. Both organizations are independent of the natural medicine industrial and sales complex and make their findings and recommendations publicly available via internet subscription.

You can also get information online from NSF®, USP®, and Labdoor about the products they have evaluated.

The Bottom Line: Be Wise and Cautious

I've adapted the cautions NCCIH gives health consumers:

- The amount of scientific evidence we have on dietary supplements varies widely—we have a lot of information on some and very little on others.

- Some dietary supplements can be good for your health; however, most have insufficient evidence that they are safe and effective.

- Legitimate peer-reviewed studies of many supplements frequently do not support claims made about them.

- Supplements you buy from stores or online often differ in important ways from products tested in studies.

- Some products marketed as dietary supplements may contain prescription drugs not allowed in dietary supplements or other ingredients not listed on the label. Some of these ingredients may be unsafe.

- The FDA does not have the resources to test all products marketed as natural medicines.
- Most shockingly of all, you cannot trust what many labels say.[35]

With these cautions understood, let's unravel the mysteries of what, if any, natural medicines you should consider for many common conditions. But first let's learn about the most effective ways to increase the quantity and quality of your remaining years.

3

What's More Effective Than *Any* Natural Medicine?

As I'll make clear throughout this book, the most effective "natural" interventions that may not only improve but also lengthen your life are not natural medicines. Rather, they are a series of healthy lifestyle habits. There is not a single natural medicine or combination of them that comes anywhere close to improving the quality and quantity of your life than choosing one or more of the following (this list is not all-inclusive):

- Drink little or no alcohol.
- Avoid tobacco products.
- Connect socially with positive relationships with family and friends.
- Eat a nutrient-dense diet, such as a Mediterranean-style or primarily plant-based diet.
- Exercise, move, and avoid a sedentary lifestyle.
- Foster mental stimulation, lifelong learning, and cognitively stimulating activities.
- Maintain a healthy blood pressure, blood sugar, cholesterol, and weight.
- Reduce stress and anxiety.

- Make restful vacations, time outdoors, quiet time, and meditation regular and routine.
- Get enough rest and sleep.
- Incorporate spirituality (particularly what I call *positive spirituality*) and prayer.

These lifestyle habits, especially when combined, may result in fairly dramatic reductions in cancer, cardiovascular disease, dementia and Alzheimer's disease, depression, and premature death. Also, they can provide mental and physical health benefits. They may increase the life expectancy of fifty-year-old people by 50 percent and cut the risk of developing Alzheimer's disease by up to 60 percent![1] In other words, they can significantly increase the likelihood of a longer and healthier life—a life that has increased quantity and quality—and who doesn't want that? These lifestyle habits are not only inexpensive and relatively risk-free, not adapting them also explains up to three-quarters of premature cardiovascular deaths and half of the premature cancer deaths in the US.[2]

In subsequent chapters in which I highlight one or more of these lifestyle interventions, I'll provide the citations from peer-reviewed medical literature that healthy habits outperform natural medicines. But I want to introduce this idea early in the book because the simple fact is that no prescription drug, over-the-counter drug, medical food (food specially formulated for the dietary management of a disease), or natural medicine (herb, vitamin, or supplement) has ever produced such profound benefits. Gad A. Marshall, MD, an assistant professor at Harvard Medical School, says, "It's wise to make as many healthy lifestyle choices as you can. They're all beneficial."[3]

A critical point is that you don't have to do them all. You certainly don't have to do them all at once. Heidi Godman, the executive editor of the *Harvard Health Letter*, explains,

> Don't feel like you need to rush into a ramped-up routine of living a healthier lifestyle. All it takes is one small change at a time, such as
>
> - exercising an extra day per week,
> - getting rid of one unhealthy food from your diet,
> - going to bed half an hour earlier or shutting off electronic gadgets a half hour earlier than usual to help wind down,

- listening to a new kind of music, or listening to a podcast about a topic you're unfamiliar with,
- or having lunch with a friend you haven't seen in a while.

Once you make one small change, try making another. Over time, they will add up. My change is that I'm going to add 15 more minutes to my exercise routine; that way, I'll rack up more exercise minutes per week, and I won't feel bad if I have to skip a workout now and then. By putting my health first, I'll be in better shape for my family and my job, and hopefully, I'll be better off in older age.[4]

If you wish to concentrate on these lifestyle changes, I've written some books to help: *10 Essentials of Happy, Healthy People: Becoming and Staying Highly Healthy*; *Fit over 50: Make Simple Choices Today for a Healthier, Happier You* (also great for younger people); and *SuperSized Kids: How to Rescue Your Child from the Obesity Threat* (also great for adults).

Should you quit reading or put this book back on the shelf? Heavens no! There are natural medicines that can add to the effectiveness of these essential habits in certain situations. My point is that you certainly can and should consider natural medications, when indicated, but not as a replacement for a foundation of healthy habits. And be sure that the natural choices you select (1) have evidence of safety *and* effectiveness and (2) have been "Certified," "Verified," or "Approved" by an independent quality testing lab such as NSF®, ConsumerLab.com, Labdoor, or USP®.

To determine your health foundation, I have developed a tool to help you assess the status of your physical, emotional, relational, and spiritual health—what I call *The Four Wheels of Health*.[5] Visit my website at DrWalt.com and scroll to the bottom of the page, where you'll see a link to "Assessment Tools and Websites." Click on either (1) "Assess Your Health—Adult Secular"[6] or (2) "Assess Your Health—Adult Christian."[7] The latter has a more robust spiritual history for Christians. It can take up to an hour to answer the questions in each assessment.

When you've completed the assessment, print the "4 Wheel Diagram—Adult."[8] Follow the simple instructions, and if you have answered all the questions honestly, you'll have an accurate visual picture of your four health wheels. Are any flat? Out of balance? In need of a tune-up? If so, I have help and hope for you!

4

Safety and Effectiveness Ratings

How They Are Determined

For the recommendation charts at the end of most chapters, I've adapted an evidence-based "Safety Rating" and "Effectiveness Rating" from *Natural Medicines*™. The charts *Natural Medicines* utilizes are just one of the many reasons I love this resource. My adaptations of their recommendations are for adults only. They are *not* ratings for breastfeeding or pregnant women or for children. However, recommendations for each of those groups are available in the *Natural Medicines* monographs that I reference for you.

Safety

Natural Medicines does not use a rating of "Safe." Their "Likely Safe" means "Safe" and that there are no safety concerns.

"Likely Safe": This product has a very high level of reliable clinical evidence showing its safe use when used appropriately. Products rated "Likely Safe" are generally considered appropriate to use as long as they are "Effective" or "Likely Effective." To achieve this safety rating, a product is supported by *all* of the following:

- Safety data are available from multiple (two or more) randomized clinical trials or meta-analysis or large-scale postmarketing surveillance, including several hundred patients (level of evidence = A). Or the product has undergone a safety review consistent with or equivalent to passing review by the FDA, Health Canada, or similarly rigorous approval process.

- Studies have a low risk of bias and a high level of validity by meeting stringent assessment criteria (quality rating = A).
- Studies adequately measure and report safety and adverse outcomes data and consistently show no significant serious adverse effects without valid evidence to the contrary.

"Possibly Safe": This product has some clinical evidence showing its safe use when used appropriately; however, the evidence is limited by quantity, quality, or contradictory findings. Products rated "Possibly Safe" appear to be safe but do not have enough high-quality evidence to recommend for most people. To achieve this safety rating, a product is supported by all of the following:

- Safety data are available from one or more randomized clinical trials, meta-analysis (level of evidence = A or B), case series, two or more population-based or epidemiological studies (level of evidence = B), or limited postmarketing surveillance data.
- Studies have a low-to-moderate risk of bias and moderate-to-high level of validity by meeting or partially meeting assessment criteria (quality rating = A or B).
- Studies adequately measure and report safety and adverse outcomes data and show no significant serious adverse effects without substantial evidence to the contrary. Some contrary evidence may exist; however, valid evidence supporting safety outweighs contrary evidence.

Effectiveness

Effectiveness ratings are assigned for specific indications. A product might be rated "Possibly Effective" for one condition but be rated "Likely Ineffective" for another condition, depending on the evidence. The evidence-based criteria for effectiveness ratings are as follows.

"Effective": This product has a very high level of reliable clinical evidence supporting its use for a specific indication. Products rated "Effective" are generally considered appropriate to recommend. To achieve this effectiveness rating, a product is supported by all of the following:

- Evidence consistent with or equivalent to passing a review by the FDA, Health Canada, or similarly rigorous approval process.
- Evidence from multiple (two or more) randomized clinical trials or meta-analysis, including several hundred to several thousand patients (level of evidence = A).
- Studies have a low risk of bias and a high level of validity by meeting stringent assessment criteria (quality rating = A).
- Evidence consistently shows positive outcomes for a given indication without valid evidence to the contrary.

"Likely Effective": This product has a very high level of reliable clinical evidence supporting its use for a specific indication. Products rated "Likely Effective" are generally considered appropriate to take. To achieve this effectiveness rating, a product is supported by all of the following:

- Evidence from multiple (two or more) randomized clinical trials or meta-analysis, including several hundred patients (level of evidence = A).
- Studies have a low risk of bias and a high level of validity by meeting stringent assessment criteria (quality rating = A).
- Evidence consistently shows positive outcomes for a given indication without significant valid evidence to the contrary.

"Possibly Effective": This product has some clinical evidence supporting its use for a specific indication; however, the evidence is limited by quantity, quality, or contradictory findings. Products rated "Possibly Effective" might be beneficial but do not have enough high-quality evidence to recommend that most people use this product. To achieve this effectiveness rating, a product is supported by all of the following:

- One or more randomized clinical trials or meta-analysis (level of evidence = A or B) or two or more population-based or epidemiological studies (level of evidence = B).
- Studies have a low-to-moderate risk of bias and moderate-to-high level of validity by meeting or partially meeting assessment criteria (quality rating = A or B).
- Evidence shows positive outcomes for a given indication without substantial valid evidence to the contrary. Some contrary evidence may exist; however, valid positive evidence outweighs contrary evidence.

Insufficient Reliable Evidence

Natural Medicines uses the designation "Insufficient Reliable Evidence," which I'll shorten to "Insufficient Evidence," when there is not enough reliable scientific evidence to provide a safety rating or an effectiveness rating. *Natural Medicines* says, "In general, people should not take products with an 'Insufficient Evidence' rating." Also, they caution, "It is important to keep in mind that different studies often use different product extracts or formulations. Results from studies using specific product formulations can only be applied to that one formulation of the product and cannot be extrapolated to other extracts or product formulations. In some cases, different study results are found when different product formulas are used." Furthermore, these ratings "assume the use of high-quality, uncontaminated products and the use of typical doses. Keep in mind that some products are never appropriate for some patients due to concomitant disease states, potential drug interactions, or other clinical factors."

Finally, I do not recommend, nor should you purchase or take, products rated by *Natural Medicines* as "Unsafe," "Likely Unsafe," "Possibly Unsafe," "Ineffective," "Likely Ineffective," or "Possibly Ineffective."

With this introductory background, let's get started on the complex, mysterious, and potentially hazardous (to your health and finances) world of natural medicines.

PART TWO

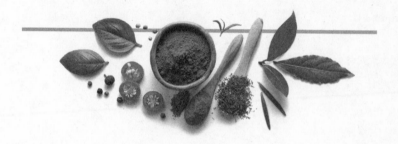

5

An Overall Approach to Wellness and Multivitamins

The National Center for Complementary and Alternative Medicine (NCCAM) once defined *complementary and alternative medicine* (CAM) as a "group of diverse medical and healthcare practices that are not generally considered to be part of conventional medicine."[1] In other words, CAM was not a part of traditional Western medicine. These terms are undergoing a dramatic evolution. *Complementary* now describes the use of nontraditional with conventional therapies. In other words, these treatments complement or augment traditional medicine. *Alternative* most often refers to the use of nontraditional or nonproven modalities instead of conventional or proven ones.

I prefer the term *integrative*, which means to combine the best of the nontraditional with the best of traditional medicine. Some use the phrase *integrative medicine*, but given that even the word *medicine* often leads people to think of pharmaceutical solutions to disease, I'm not as comfortable using this term. I think many people prefer, as I do, to think of "health and healing" instead of "medicine"; therefore, I often use the phrase *integrative health and healing*.

In my practice, teaching, and writing, I use and recommend only therapies, modalities, medications, interventions, and approaches that are *both* safe and effective, ones more likely to help than harm a person's body, mind, spirit, *and* wallet. I also emphasize the importance of physical, emotional/ mental, relational/social, and spiritual health. I call these "the four wheels of health." Thousands of medical studies have confirmed the intricate interconnection between each of them. If one or more of your four wheels of health are flat or out of balance, your ride in life is likely to be more uncomfortable, and if a wheel has an unexpected blowout, your journey is suddenly bumpier and shorter.

When sickness or illness comes, as it does to us all, I believe that every intervention offered you should aim not only to treat the disease but also to enhance your overall health and wellness. In other words, a holistic treatment should not only effectively treat the disorder but also

- improve your sense of general well-being and mental alertness,
- balance your immune system to protect from illness, and
- improve your physical, emotional, relational, and spiritual health and wellness.

Increasing Quality and Quantity of Life

The National Wellness Institute expands on my four wheels of health analogy and promotes "Six Dimensions of Wellness": emotional, occupational, physical, social, intellectual, and spiritual. The institute writes, "Addressing all six dimensions of wellness in our lives builds a holistic sense of wellness and fulfillment."[2] Among wellness experts, there seems to be general agreement that "wellness

- is a conscious, self-directed, and evolving process of achieving full potential,
- is multidimensional and holistic, encompassing lifestyle, mental, and spiritual well-being, and the environment, and
- is positive and affirming."[3]

Although healing and wellness are laudable goals, they are much easier to acclaim than to achieve. One reason conventional medicine and healthcare professionals tend to focus on treating diseases rather than increasing wellness is because it is easier to accomplish. Furthermore, in the not-too-distant past, many people, including health professionals, have believed the most influential force affecting wellness was genetics. As one review stated, "Many researchers have long argued that most chronic diseases are caused by humans' genetic predisposition for a condition."[4] As a result, "If a disease is thought to be caused solely by genetics, people may develop notions of fatalism and not alter their health-related behaviors."[5] In other words, some ask, "Why fight heredity?"

However, about ten years ago, experts discovered that as much as 80 percent of what controls the quantity and quality of lifespan is related to lifestyle decisions and *not* our genes, which only accounted for about 20 percent of an individual's chance of surviving and thriving into old age.[6] Then, a 2018 study in the journal *Genetics*, published by the Genetics Society of America, reported that "genes accounted for well under seven percent of people's life span."[7]

Genes are important, but even *more* essential are the decisions *you* make about daily lifestyle issues—sleeping, diet, exercise, work, leisure, meditation, prayer, smoking, drug use or abuse, reducing stress, and improving relationships. That's why physicians and wellness experts who practice evidence-based healthcare are increasingly stressing that people with almost any chronic disease emphasize enhancing their lifestyle. The goal is to prevent illness before treatment is even needed.

One great example is in the area of healthy nutrition. Researchers from the Harvard T.H. Chan School of Public Health write, "A diet rich in vegetables and fruits can

- lower blood pressure,
- reduce the risk of heart disease and stroke,
- prevent some types of cancer,
- lower risk of eye and digestive problems, and
- have a positive effect upon blood sugar, which can help keep appetite in check."

They add, "Eating nonstarchy vegetables and fruits like apples, pears, and green leafy vegetables may even promote weight loss. Their low glycemic loads prevent blood sugar spikes that can increase hunger."[8] A 2014 review of sixteen studies involving more than 833,000 people reported that those who consumed five servings of fruits and vegetables a day lowered their risk of dying from heart disease by 20 percent compared with those who consumed fewer servings.[9]

In 2018, Harvard researchers reported their evaluation of five healthy habits:

1. Never smoking
2. Maintaining a normal weight BMI of 18.5 to 24.9
3. Thirty or more minutes per day of moderate-to-vigorous physical activity
4. No or limited alcohol intake
5. A high-quality, primarily plant-based, whole-foods, nutrient-dense diet[10]

Their findings were astounding. Fifty-year-old women who followed all five habits lived an average of fourteen years longer than women who did not. For men it was twelve years of additional life expectancy.[11] That's about a 50 percent increase!

But, you may say, why live longer if there's no quality to my life? Great question! The same research team looked at quality-of-life issues and reported their startling findings in 2020. Senior author Frank Hu, MD, PhD, a professor of medicine at Harvard Medical School, told CNN, "Following a healthy lifestyle can substantially extend the years a person lives disease-free."[12]

But what if I've smoked in the past? Or what if I'm overweight? What if only four of the five healthy habits are possible for me? In that case, Dr. Hu and his team have more great news: "Women who practiced four or five of the healthy habits over the next 20 to 30 years," Hu said, "had an additional 10.6 years of disease-free living compared to women who adopted no lifestyle changes. When broken down by disease, the healthier women gained an average of 8 years free of cancer, 10 years with no cardiovascular disease, and 12 years without diabetes." He added, "Men who practiced four to five healthy behaviors gained 7.6 years' longer life expectancy; an average of 6 more years without cancer, almost 9 more years free of heart issues, and over 10 years without diabetes."[13]

CNN asked, "What happened if a person was diagnosed with a disease during the study?" Dr. Hu responded, "The data showed half of people diagnosed with cancer lived an additional 23 years if they adopted four of five healthy practices. Among those who didn't change, half only survived an additional 11 years. The same patterns were seen for both heart disease and diabetes." Dr. Hu added, "This is a positive health message because it means healthy lifestyle habits not only prolong life but also improve the quality of life and reduce sufferings related to chronic diseases."[14]

If you're a smoker, stopping has impressive benefits. It's never too late to stop using tobacco. Furthermore, the sooner you quit, the more you can reduce your chances of getting cancer and other diseases. According to the American Cancer Society (ACS):

- Twenty minutes after quitting, your heart rate and blood pressure drop.
- Twelve hours after quitting, the carbon monoxide level in your blood drops to normal.
- Two weeks to three months after quitting, your circulation improves, and your lung function increases.
- One to nine months after quitting, coughing and shortness of breath decrease.
- One year after quitting, the excess risk of coronary heart disease is half that of someone who still smokes. Your heart attack risk drops dramatically.
- Two to five years after quitting, your stroke risk can fall to that of a nonsmoker.
- Five years after quitting, your risk of cancers of the mouth, throat, esophagus, and bladder is cut in half; cervical cancer risk falls to that of a nonsmoker.

- Ten years after quitting, your risk of dying from lung cancer is about half that of a person who is still smoking; your risk of cancer of the larynx (voice box) and pancreas decreases.
- Fifteen years after quitting, your risk of coronary heart disease is that of a nonsmoker.[15]

Kicking the tobacco habit also offers some very pleasant rewards that you'll notice right away:

- Immediately you'll save the money you spent on tobacco!
- Food tastes better, and your sense of smell returns to normal.
- Your breath, hair, and clothes smell better.
- Your teeth and fingernails stop yellowing.
- Quitting also helps stop the damaging effects of tobacco on how you look, including premature wrinkling of your skin, gum disease, and tooth loss.[16]

What about vaping or e-cigarettes? According to the ACS, "E-cigarettes, or 'vaping,' are terms used synonymously to refer to the use of a wide variety of electronic, battery-operated devices that aerosolize, but do not burn, liquids to release nicotine and other substances." Are these safe to use, or should they be used to help one stop smoking? The ACS says, "All tobacco products, including e-cigarettes [or vaping], pose a risk to the health of the user. . . . The long-term risks of exclusive use of e-cigarettes are not fully known, but evidence is accumulating that e-cigarette use has negative effects on the cardiovascular system and lungs." They add, "The ACS does not recommend the use of e-cigarettes as a cessation method. No e-cigarette has been approved by the Food and Drug Administration (FDA) as a safe and effective cessation product."[17]

Spirituality

In regard to lifestyle health benefits, Harold G. Koenig, MD, the senior fellow in the Center for the Study of Aging and Human Development at Duke University, reviewed hundreds of research reports that examined the relationship between religion/spirituality (R/S) and health. He writes, "A large volume of research shows that people who are more religious/spiritual have better mental health and adapt more quickly to health problems compared to those who are less religious/spiritual. These possible benefits to mental health and well-being have physiological consequences that impact physical health, affect the risk of disease, and influence response to treatment."[18]

For both overall wellness and "positive aging," researchers now have found that "religion, spirituality, or belief . . . play a number of roles in the everyday lives of adults, including being a source of strength, comfort and hope in difficult times, and bringing about a sense of community and belonging."[19] FamilyDoctor.org writes, "Research shows a connection between your beliefs and your sense of well-being. Positive beliefs, comfort, and strength gained from religion, meditation, and prayer can contribute to well-being. It may even promote healing. Improving your spiritual health may . . . prevent some health problems and help you cope better with illness, stress, or death."[20]

The Bible reminds us, "Physical training is of some value, but godliness has value for all things, holding promise for both the present life and the life to come."[21] I join the apostle John in saying to you, "Dear friend, I pray that you may enjoy good health and that all may go well with you, even as your soul is getting along well."[22]

By far, the most significant impact on your overall wellness involves your health habits—what you do, *not* what natural medicines you take. This is even more important when you consider that, according to the *Natural and Alternative Treatments*™ *Encyclopedia*, "no natural (medicines) have been proven effective for enhancing overall wellness."[23] No, not one!

Nevertheless, the public has not picked up this message, and as a result, "overall wellness" is the number one reason people use natural medicines, particularly multivitamins.[24] Is this a wise and good economic decision? Let's examine the evidence. I bet you'll be surprised.

Multivitamins—Not Healthy or Helpful?

In 2019, US multivitamin sales totaled more than $7.56 billion, a 3.2 percent increase compared with the same period the previous year.[25] This is about

18 percent of the $46.2 billion sales of all dietary supplements in the US.[26] One 2019 national survey reported a majority of adults take vitamins—mostly to "maintain health and prevent disease."[27] Another national analysis found multivitamins were the most commonly used supplement—taken by 71 percent of people. The reason most often cited for multivitamin use was "overall health and wellness" (58 percent).[28]

Johns Hopkins researchers reported that "70 percent of those age sixty-five and older take a multivitamin . . . regularly." They advise that this money would be "far better spent on nutrient-packed foods like fruit, vegetables, whole grains, and low-fat dairy products."[29] In an editorial in the journal *Annals of Internal Medicine* titled "Enough Is Enough: Stop Wasting Money on Vitamin and Mineral Supplements," Johns Hopkins experts reviewed the evidence about multivitamins from three sizeable and well-performed studies:

- An analysis of 450,000 people found that multivitamins did not reduce the risk for heart disease or cancer.
- A study that tracked 5,947 men for twelve years found that multivitamins did not reduce the risk for mental declines such as memory loss or slowed-down thinking.
- A study of 1,708 heart attack survivors who took a high-dose multivitamin or placebo for up to fifty-five months reported that the rates of later heart attacks, heart surgeries, and deaths were similar in both groups.

The Johns Hopkins experts concluded that "multivitamins don't reduce the risk for heart disease, cancer, cognitive decline (such as memory loss and slowed-down thinking), or early death. . . . The studies published in this issue and previous trials indicate no substantial health benefit. . . . (Yet) sales of multivitamins have not been affected by major studies with null results."[30]

This conclusion agrees with a 2018 review of the literature in the *Journal of the American College of Cardiology*, which found that multivitamins did not lower the risk of heart disease, stroke, or premature death.[31] In 2019 Tufts University researchers reported their evaluation of more than twenty-seven thousand US adults age twenty or older who answered questions about their dietary supplement use and their diets. More than half reported using at least one supplement, and more than one-third used a multivitamin. The researchers found that specific vitamins and minerals were associated with a lower risk of premature death from heart disease or stroke and an overall lower risk of dying during the average six years of follow-up. But these findings were valid *only* when the nutrients came from foods, *not* from supplements! Furthermore, the study found that consuming high levels of calcium from supplements—at least 1,000 milligrams per day—was linked to a higher risk of death from cancer. However, there was no link between intake of calcium from food and the risk of death from cancer.[32]

"It's pretty clear that vitamin and supplement use has no benefit for the general population. They are not a substitute for a healthy balanced diet," said Fang Fang Zhang, PhD, a professor at the Friedman School of Nutrition Science and Policy at Tufts and the study's senior author.[33] In another interview, Dr. Zhang added, "Our findings suggest that adequate nutrient intake from foods was associated with reduced mortality, [while] excess intake from [multivitamin] supplements could be harmful."[34]

This study wasn't the first to link supplement use with harmful effects. In 2011, a large study found that use of vitamin E supplements was connected to an increased risk of prostate cancer in men.[35] That year, a separate study among older women found that use of multivitamin supplements was related to an increased risk of premature death during the twenty-year study period.[36] An extensive 2016 review concluded, "Taking supplements of vitamin E, A, C, D, and folic acid [vitamin B9] for prevention of disease or cancer is not effective and can even be harmful to the health. So, it would be rational to limit these supplements consumption to those having deficiencies of the mentioned vitamins."[37]

Finally, a massive 2019 analysis encompassing 277 studies of nearly one million people concluded, "Vitamins, minerals, dietary supplements, and dietary interventions were not associated with survival or cardiovascular benefits." Furthermore, they found the combined use of taking calcium and vitamin D supplements increased the risk for stroke seventeen percent.[38]

In 2019, *Natural Medicines*™ reviewed the best studies on multivitamin use from around the world and determined that "the available evidence is that multivitamins are not effective for the prevention of Alzheimer disease, cardiovascular disease, overall mortality, or stroke." Furthermore, they add, there is "Insufficient Evidence" to take them "for the prevention of cancer, decreased cognitive function, or stress." Dr. Meredith Worthington says, "For this reason, *Natural Medicines* recommends that people NOT take multivitamins for these indications."

The Dietary Guidelines for Americans 2015–2020, developed by nutrition and health experts from the US Department of Health and Human Services (HHS) and the US Department of Agriculture (USDA), recommend that "people should aim to meet their nutrient requirements through a healthy eating pattern that includes nutrient-dense forms of foods."[39] Nutrient-dense foods are high in nutrients but relatively low in calories. Better yet, they contain vitamins, minerals, complex carbohydrates, lean protein, and healthy fats. Examples of nutrient-dense foods include fruits and vegetables, whole grains, low-fat or fat-free milk products, seafood, lean meats, eggs, peas, beans, and nuts.[40]

The Academy of Nutrition and Dietetics (AND), the largest organization of food and nutrition professionals in the US (representing over one hundred thousand credentialed professionals), agrees and recommends that people try to get their nutrients from foods by eating a healthy diet that includes nutrient-dense foods and not through vitamins or supplements. The AND points out that "foods can contain beneficial components that aren't found in supplements, such as fiber or bioactive compounds."[41] The US Preventive Services Task Force (USPSTF), an independent panel of experts that develops recommendations for clinical preventive services, concluded in 2019 that there simply isn't sufficient evidence to recommend the use of multivitamins for cancer or cardiovascular disease prevention.[42]

Lastly, the FDA reported in 2019 that large, hard multivitamin and calcium supplements were a frequent cause of choking in seniors—accounting for 19 percent of all reported adverse events with natural medicines from 2006 to 2015. Multivitamins were the most dangerous, accounting for almost 73 percent of the reports. The size of generic or branded prescription products is strictly limited. But natural medicines are not subject to such scrutiny.[43] ConsumerLab gives the size of the pills it rates.

Some people *do* benefit from multivitamins—for example, people with specific diseases (such as celiac disease or other malabsorptive conditions, chronic kidney disease, patients who've undergone gastric bypass, or those with age-related macular degeneration), people using specific medications (such as anti-seizure drugs or bile acid sequestrants), and specific groups (such as pregnant women and the elderly).

However, most adults who eat nutritious foods such as fruits, vegetables, legumes, and whole grains along with heart-healthy fats and lean protein will not need a multivitamin, as their diet will provide all the vitamins and minerals they need. Nevertheless, if your healthcare professional recommends a multivitamin for a specific purpose, you need to be careful which one you purchase, as there are significant quality issues with nonprescription multivitamins.

Multivitamins—If You Buy, Which Do You Buy?

In a 2020 review, ConsumerLab.com reported testing thirty-five popular multivitamin/multimineral supplements, including products for seniors, men, women (including prenatal vitamins), diabetics, children, and pets. They found that nine "failed to gain our approval because we discovered much lower or higher amounts of vitamins or minerals than listed on their labels or they took too long to fully break apart." In other words, of the thirty-five, 74 percent (26) were ConsumerLab "Approved," while the nine products (26%) that failed one or more quality tests were "Not Approved." Of concern to me, 60 percent of men's vitamins" (three of five) and 66 percent of prenatal vitamins (two of three) failed one or more tests and were "Not Approved." As an aside, they tested four vitamin products for pets. Three of the four were "Not Approved."

ConsumerLab noted, "Of particular concern is that several products provided more than or close to the Upper Tolerable Intake Levels (ULs), above which there is increasing risk of toxicity with regular use." As with their previous tests of multivitamins, they found, "Most gummy formulations did not contain the listed amounts of nutrients—having far less or far more."

ConsumerLab's "Top Picks" for 2020 include:

- General Adult: *"Kirkland Signature*™ [Costco®] *Daily Multi* which "provided at least 100 percent of the recommended daily intake of many vitamins and minerals without exceeding any upper tolerable intake levels (ULs) and cost just 3 cents per day per tablet—far less than other multivitamins."

- Adult 50+: *Equate*™ [Walmart] *Complete Multivitamin 50+* (3 cents per daily tablet) or *Up & Up*™ [Target] *Adults 50+ Multivitamin* (4 cents per daily tablet) as well as *Centrum® Silver®* "which we tested and 'Approved' in 2017 but cost more (8 cents per daily tablet)."

- Women's: *Bayer One A Day® Women's Formula* (11 cents per daily tablet). They add, *"Up & Up*™ [Target] *Women's Daily Multivitamin*, which was 'Approved' in our tests in 2017, is essentially identical in formulation and costs only 3 cents per tablet —less than one-third the price of Bayer."

- Women's 50+: *Bayer One A Day® Women's 50+* (14 cents per daily tablet).

- Prenatal: *Deva® Prenatal One Daily* (12 cents per daily tablet).

- Men's: *Nature Made® Men's Multi* (15 cents per daily softgel).

- Men's 50+: *Member's Mark* [Sam's Club®] *Men 50+ Multivitamin* (3 cents per daily tablet).

ConsumerLab advises, "If you have trouble swallowing large pills, consider a chewable vitamin, but not a gummy." This year they "Approved" *Centrum® Silver® Chewables Adults 50+ Citrus Berry* (27 cents per daily chewable).

When defining multivitamins as products containing three or more vitamins or minerals (and no herbs), *Natural Medicines* lists about 117 that are NMBER® rated 8 out of 10 or above. USP® has "Verified" thirty-seven vitamins and twenty-two multivitamins, including products from *Kirkland Signature*™ and *Nature Made®*. Labdoor gave two multivitamins a "Certified for Sport" rating, two a "B" rating, and another eleven a "B-minus" rating, including products from *Garden of Life®*, *Nature's Way®*, and GNC (I only recommend "A" and "B" rated products from Labdoor).[44] NSF® has "Certified" eight multivitamin products.[45]

But, once again, unless recommended by your health professional for a specific indication, multivitamins are no longer advised for the average adult.

Other Natural Medicines for Wellness

Are there other natural medicines for wellness? The short answer is that there's nothing I can recommend. Researchers writing in the *Annals of Internal Medicine* agree: "Evidence is sufficient to advise against routine supplementation" with natural medications for wellness or disease prevention. "The message is simple: most supplements do not prevent chronic disease or death, their use is not justified, and they should be avoided. This message is especially true for the general population with no clear evidence of micronutrient deficiencies, who represent most supplement users in the US and in other countries."[46]

The Bottom Line: The *Best* Way to Live

Francis Collins, MD, PhD, the director of the NIH and the former director of the Human Genome Project, writes, "Right now, the best way to live a long and healthy life is to follow the good advice offered by the rigorous and highly objective reviews provided by the US Preventive Services Task Force. Those tend to align with what I hope your parents offered: eat a balanced diet, including plenty of fruits, veggies, and healthy sources of calcium and protein. Don't smoke. Use alcohol in moderation. Avoid recreational drugs. Get plenty of exercise."[47]

Dr. Collins also adds, "But a purely materialist approach, stripping away the spiritual aspect of humanity, will impoverish us—after all, that has been already tried (in Stalin's USSR and Mao's China) and found to be devastating. . . . I try to spend time in prayer in the morning while the world is still quiet. But I also try to keep my spiritual side awake and alert during the day. . . . I am still working on deepening my relationship with God, and that is a lifelong task."[48]

I would agree.

Although I do not have the space to discuss the many other natural medicines that people push and peddle for overall wellness, I've included ratings of the more common ones in the following chart. More detailed information is available from ConsumerLab.com and *Natural Medicines*.

Natural Interventions and Medications for Overall Wellness

Effective \ Safe	Likely Safe	Possibly Safe
Effective	★★★★★ • Avoid tobacco products • Nutrient-dense foods (fruits, vegetables, lean protein, heart-healthy fats) • Regular exercise • Restful sleep • Stop smoking	★★★
Likely Effective	★★★★ • Avoid social isolation • Fiber-rich diet • Maintain a normal BMI • Mental stimulation • Nurture friendships • Prayer, meditation, positive spirituality • Reduce stress	★★
Possibly Effective	★★★ • Cultivate life's "wow" moments	★ • Alcohol (beer/wine) in moderation
Insufficient evidence for safety or effectiveness AND/OR evidence for lack of safety or effectiveness		
 • Calcium supplements • Dietary supplements • Herbal products • Mineral supplements • Multivitamins		

Most of the recommendations in the chart are based on the "Safety and Effectiveness Ratings" contained in *Natural Medicines™* and explained in chapter 4 of this book. They assume the use of high-quality, uncontaminated products and the use of typical doses. Keep in mind that some products are never appropriate for some patients due to concomitant disease states, potential drug interactions, or other clinical factors. Details are available at *Natural Medicines™*.

6

Brain Health—Part 1

Individual Natural Medicines

Let me begin this chapter with the bottom line: no prescription drug, over-the-counter drug, medical food, or natural medicine (herb, vitamin, or supplement) has ever produced a clear benefit for helping preserve memory or for preventing Alzheimer's disease (AD) or any other form of dementia. The experts at *Natural Medicines*™ write, "There is no therapy to slow the natural cognitive decline that occurs with aging." Let's look at some basics and then dig into the details.

Aging (yes, even when we're very young) is associated with changes in brain structure and function. But starting about age forty, brain change accelerates. Brain volume and weight decrease at a rate of approximately 5 percent every ten years. The speed of loss increases after age seventy. Memory loss is a common and normal complaint that typically starts between the ages of forty and fifty.[1] The old joke is that normal age-related memory loss is forgetting where you put your keys. Abnormal is not remembering what they are used for.

Besides declines in working memory, other cognitive changes that occur after age fifty are a steady slow loss in our speed of processing information (e.g., making a decision) and a concomitant decrease in executive functioning ability (the brain-based skills of goal setting and self-regulation).[2]

Dementia

Dementia is the overarching term for a family of progressive brain diseases that slowly destroys memory and thinking skills. There is a spectrum from normal age-related memory loss to several forms of dementia, including Alzheimer's disease, which is the most common form of dementia. AD is 100 percent fatal, the only top-ten cause of death in the US with *no* known cure, and the third leading cause of death after heart disease and cancer. No wonder AD is "the most feared disease in the US."[3]

In a 2019 survey, almost half of Americans in their fifties and sixties believed they were at least "somewhat likely" to develop dementia—even though "the estimated proportion of the general population ages sixty and over with dementia at a given time is only five to eight percent."[4] Nevertheless, a US survey found almost one-in-three adults (31 percent) identified AD as their most feared illness when presented with a list of health issues, including cancer, stroke, heart disease, and diabetes.[5] In another poll, six times as many older people were more fearful of developing dementia than they were of cancer.[6] On top of that, people increasingly understand there are no medical cures for AD.

As a result, more and more consumers are buying into the hype surrounding natural medicines to either prevent brain decline or improve brain health. The FDA estimated that "eighty percent of older adults rely on dietary supplements, many purporting to prevent or treat Alzheimer's and other forms of dementia."[7]

The 2019 AARP® Brain Health and Dietary Supplements Survey reported that "more than a quarter of Americans age fifty and older are regularly taking . . . at least one supplement for brain-health reasons. Among adults specifically taking dietary supplements for brain health, about half take dietary supplements to maintain—and the other half to improve—their brain health."[8] Another survey reported one-third or more of adults were taking supplements to help ward off memory decline.[9] As a result, the sales of supplements claiming to boost memory have nearly doubled from 2006 to 2015. In 2016, sales of brain-health supplements totaled $3 billion. That's projected to increase to $5.8 billion by 2023.[10]

Unfortunately, almost all of these concerned and fearful people are wasting their money.

Cochrane is a global independent network of researchers and professionals. Many are world leaders in their fields. They work together to produce credible, accessible health information that is free from commercial sponsorship and other conflicts of interest.[11] In 2018 they published a review of every study evaluating vitamin or mineral supplements for preventing dementia or delaying mild cognitive impairment (MCI). They concluded, "It is not possible to identify any supplements which can reduce the risk of people with MCI developing dementia or which can effectively treat their symptoms."[12] Mayo Clinic neurologist David S. Knopman, MD, a researcher in dementia and Alzheimer's, agrees, saying, "There is zero evidence from any reasonably rigorous study that any supplement or dietary aid has any benefit on cognitive function or decline in late life."[13]

In 2018, AARP® became so concerned about this issue that they formed the Global Council on Brain Health (GCBH)—an independent collaborative of scientists, health professionals, scholars, and policy experts from around the world who are working in areas of brain health related to human cognition. In their exhaustive 2019 report, they advised, "We do not endorse any ingredient, product, or supplement formulation specifically for brain health unless your health care provider has identified that you have a specific nutrient deficiency."[14] Journalist Kathleen Fifield reported, "The report analyzes existing studies on supplements that purport to boost cognition—from fish oil to apoaequorin (a protein from jellyfish), with the authors finding insufficient evidence to recommend any type of supplement for brain health for most adults."[15] AARP® added: "GCBH does not recommend *any* dietary supplement for brain health."[16]

No, not one. There are no natural medicines that help. Nada. Naught. Nothing. Zilch. Zero. So should you skip this chapter? No! Heaven forbid! Because there *is* help and hope available for you and your family. Kirsty Marais from Alzheimer's Research UK says that one of the most common questions put to them is "How can I prevent dementia?"[17] And here is how.

Lifestyle Habits and Brain Health

It is well-known that both genetic and lifestyle factors play a role in determining individual risk of dementia and Alzheimer's disease. However, any genetic risk you may have could be offset by lifestyle factors.[18] Daniel L. Murman, MD, the director of the Memory Disorders Program at the University of Nebraska, writes, "There is emerging evidence that healthy lifestyle choices improve [brain health]." He specifically mentions the following:

- eating a healthy diet
- avoiding excessive alcohol consumption
- exercising regularly
- participating in cognitive-stimulating activities
- managing emotional stress, which might include meditation
- managing medical problems, such as hypertension, diabetes, depression, and obstructive sleep apnea[19]

The Lancet Commission on Dementia listed nine "modifiable risk factors" for dementia—things that we can do something about—including smoking, lack of physical activity, and social isolation.[20]

A healthy lifestyle cuts your risk of developing Alzheimer's disease[21] by up to 60 percent.[22] It can also dramatically reduce your risk of other forms of dementia even if you have genes that raise your risk for these mind-destroying diseases. British researchers found, "Regardless of how much genetic risk someone had, a good diet, adequate exercise, limiting alcohol, and not smoking made dementia less likely."[23] John Haaga, PhD, of the US National Institute on Aging said, "I consider that good news. No one can guarantee you'll escape this awful disease, but you can tip the odds in your favor with clean living."[24]

According to the *Harvard Health Letter*, "so far, evidence suggests that several healthy habits may help ward off Alzheimer's":

- *Exercise*. "The recommendation is thirty minutes of moderately vigorous aerobic exercise, three to four days per week."
- *Eat a Mediterranean diet*. "This has been shown to help thwart Alzheimer's or slow its progression. A recent study showed that even partial adherence to such a diet is better than nothing."
- *Get enough sleep*. "Growing evidence suggests that improved sleep can help prevent Alzheimer's. Aim for seven to eight hours per night."[25]

A 2019 study reported that personalized lifestyle interventions not only stopped cognitive decline in people at risk for Alzheimer's, but also increased their memory and thinking skills within eighteen months. "Our data actually shows cognitive improvement," neurologist Richard Isaacson, MD, the founder of the Alzheimer's Prevention Clinic at New York-Presbyterian and Weill Cornell Medical Center, told CNN. He added, "This is the first study in a real-world clinic setting showing individualized clinical management may improve cognitive function and also reduce Alzheimer's and cardiovascular risk." What were the two most important interventions? "Physical activity and nutrition were by far the two most important things on the list, but those were also personalized for each individual," Isaacson said.[26]

In 2020, two studies reported that risk for cognitive impairment could be reduced by half by closely follow the Mediterranean diet. Dr. Emily Chew, who directs the Division of Epidemiology and Clinical Applications (DECA) at the National Eye Institute in Bethesda, Maryland, told CNN, "People with the higher adherence to the Mediterranean diet had a 45 percent to 50 percent reduction in the risk of having an impaired cognitive function." Closely following the diet was defined as "eating fish twice a week, as well as regularly consuming fruits, vegetables, whole grains, nuts, legumes, and olive oil while reducing consumption of red meat and alcohol." High fish and vegetable consumption were associated with the greatest protective effect. In reviewing the studies, Dr. Isaacson said, "The evidence continues to mount that you are what you eat when it comes to brain health."[27]

Also, in 2020 it was reported that the high-quality "MIND" diet (Mediterranean-DASH Diet Intervention for Neurodegenerative Delay), when combined with other healthy lifestyle factors, was associated with a significantly decreased risk of Alzheimer's dementia. This conclusion was based upon studies following over twenty-five hundred older Americans for about six years.[28]

The MIND diet score is based on an evaluation of how much food is consumed in either healthy food groups (leafy green vegetables, other vegetables, nuts, berries, beans, whole grains, fish, poultry, olive oil, and wine) or less-healthy food groups (red meats, butter and stick margarine, cheese, pastries and sweets, fried food, and fast food). The more of the former and the less of the latter, the higher the score. The five healthy lifestyle factors considered were

1. having the highest MIND diet score (upper 40 percent),
2. not smoking,
3. engaging in >150 minutes per week of moderate- to vigorous-intensity physical activity,
4. light to moderate alcohol consumption (one drink per day for women and two for men), and
5. engagement in late-life cognitive activities (such as reading, writing, or playing chess).

The risk of Alzheimer's dementia was 37 percent lower in those with two to three healthy lifestyle factors and 60 percent lower in those with four to five factors compared to those with no or only one healthy lifestyle factor.

Adopting healthy lifestyle habits is not only effective but also a relatively inexpensive and risk-free way to increase both the quality and quantity of your years. Healthy living prevents or significantly delays chronic diseases such as dementia, Alzheimer's, cardiovascular disease, and cancer. Unhealthy habits (particularly the five harmful habits of smoking, not exercising, being overweight, drinking too much alcohol, and eating an unhealthy diet) significantly increase your risk of premature death and explain up to three-quarters of premature cardiovascular deaths and half of the premature cancer deaths in the US.[29]

Brain Supplements (Nootropics) in General

Harvard researchers reported, "Brain enhancement supplements [also called *nootropics*] have become increasingly popular. . . . Despite their popularity, the risks of these products are poorly understood."[30] Steven DeKosky, MD, deputy director of the McKnight Brain Institute at the University of Florida, says, "We see plenty of ads on TV, but we have no evidence that any of these things (vitamins, various antioxidants, concoctions derived from animals and plants) are preventive (of dementia or Alzheimer's)."

Moreover, he adds, "Some of these supplements are biologically active and can cause toxicity when you take other drugs."[31]

Jacob Hall, MD, a neurologist at Stanford University, writes, "There's a lot of fear and desperation surrounding memory loss and the lack of effective medications to prevent or slow it down. Supplement companies are aware of this chasm and are increasingly rushing to fill it."[32] Alzforum, a news website and information resource dedicated to helping researchers of Alzheimer's disease and related disorders, reports, "Researchers . . . believe such supplements offer false hope while shrinking the wallets of people worried about cognitive decline and dementia."[33] The FDA agrees, writing, "Simply put, health fraud scams prey on vulnerable populations, waste money, and often delay proper medical care."[34]

Neuroscientists contacted by Alzforum "universally believe brain health supplements are ineffective."[35] Paul Aisen, MD, an expert in Alzheimer's disease research and director of the Alzheimer's Therapeutic Research Institute at the University of Southern California, told Alzforum, "It is very likely that all such remedies are useless, and some are potentially hazardous."[36] The Alzheimer's Association notes that even if a supplement is safe to take on its own, it may interact with prescription medicines or other supplements in unpredictable ways.[37]

Dr. Knopman adds, "My take is that the extent of false claims made by many supplement or memory-enhancing drug manufacturers is criminal."[38] It appears the FDA agrees. In 2019, the agency mailed letters to seventeen companies formally accusing them of illegally marketing dietary supplements for dementia prevention or treatment. The supplements included vitamins, minerals, and herbal products. Some had been investigated for dementia or Alzheimer's treatments and found in large trials to be unsafe or ineffective. The FDA has issued more than forty warning letters in the past five years to companies illegally marketing over eighty products making Alzheimer's or dementia disease claims on websites, social media, and in stores.[39] Unfortunately, they're just playing Whac-A-Mole—every time they knock one down, more pop up!

Nevertheless, following is the evidence, or more accurately, lack thereof, on some of the more popular ingredients often found in products sold for brain health.

Brain Supplements (Nootropics)—Specific Substances

ACETYL-L-CARNITINE (sometimes found in stores as L-acetylcarnitine or LAC) is, according to *Natural Medicines*, "a natural medicine that has been evaluated for slowing age-related cognitive decline. . . . Taking acetyl-L-carnitine 1,500 to 2,000 mg by mouth daily for three months seems to improve some measures of cognitive function and memory in elderly people with age-related mental impairment." They add, "Acetyl-L-carnitine is generally well tolerated." However, the experts at *Natural Medicines* conclude, "Although it looks promising, it is too early to recommend acetyl-L-carnitine for slowing age-related cognitive decline. . . . Also, healthcare professionals should be aware that acetyl-L-carnitine may interact with some drugs commonly used by older patients."

ANTIOXIDANTS: BETA-CAROTENE, VITAMIN C, or VITAMIN E. A Cochrane review concludes, "The results are mixed, but the review authors say that long-term supplementation with antioxidant vitamins may be the most promising area for future research."[40]

Beta-carotene is rated as "Possibly Ineffective" for AD and as having "Insufficient Evidence" for cognitive performance by *Natural Medicines*. Furthermore, it is "Possibly Unsafe" in smokers.

Vitamin C is classified by *Natural Medicines* as "Likely Safe" but has "Insufficient Evidence" for AD or vascular dementia.

Vitamin E is rated by *Natural Medicines* as "Likely Safe" and "Possibly Effective" in treating but not preventing AD. There is "Insufficient Evidence" to treat dementia with vitamin E. Furthermore, it is "Possibly Unsafe" when used in doses exceeding 1,000 mg daily, which can be associated with significant side effects. In addition, vitamin E above 400 IU/day has been linked with increased mortality.[41]

Remember that *Natural Medicines*' "Possibly Effective" rating does not mean *Natural Medicines* would recommend a substance. It just means "this product has some clinical evidence supporting its use for a specific indication; however, the evidence is limited by quantity, quality, or contradictory findings. Products rated 'Possibly Effective' might be beneficial, but do not have enough high-quality evidence to recommend for most people."

B VITAMINS. In a 2015 review, Cochrane advised, "B vitamins have not fared any better." They found that supplementation with B6 (pyridoxine),

B12 (cobalamin), or folic acid (B9)—whether combined together or taken individually—"failed to slow or reduce the risk of cognitive decline in healthy older adults and did not improve brain function in those with cognitive decline or dementia."[42] In a 2018 update, they added, "Only B vitamins have been assessed in more than one RCT [randomized controlled trial]. There is no evidence for beneficial effects on cognition of supplementation with B vitamins for six to 24 months."[43]

Vitamin B6 (pyridoxine) is rated by *Natural Medicines* as "Possibly Ineffective" for age-related cognitive decline and to prevent or treat AD.

Vitamin B9 (folic acid) had "Insufficient Evidence" to prevent or treat AD and is "Possibly Ineffective" alone or in combination with other B vitamins in preventing or treating age-related cognitive decline.

Vitamin B12 (cobalamin) is rated as having "Insufficient Evidence" for preventing or treating AD and as "Possibly Ineffective" in improving cognition in young or elderly adults.

Taking vitamin B12 with folic acid is rated by *Natural Medicines* as "Effective" in treating any memory loss associated with a *documented deficiency* in either but not in preventing memory loss. GCBH agrees.[44]

CAFFEINE. One group of researchers writes, "Nonhuman studies suggest a protective effect of caffeine on cognition. Although human studies remain less consistent, reviews suggest a possible favorable relationship between caffeine consumption and cognitive impairment or dementia." This group studied about sixty-five hundred women ages sixty-five to eighty years and reported those consuming more than 260 mg of daily caffeine were significantly less likely to develop dementia or any cognitive impairment.[45]

Another study of older women reported that more than 371 mg of daily caffeine was associated with slower rates of cognitive decline. Of interest, these researchers found this effect in caffeinated coffee consumption but not other caffeinated products (e.g., tea, cola, or chocolate).[46]

Natural Medicines concludes, "While these preliminary results are of interest, higher quality clinical evidence is needed before caffeine can be recommended for slowing age-related cognitive decline." As an aside, caffeine intake, especially in doses over 400 mg daily, is not advised for any adult. For more information about caffeine, see the appendix.

FISH OIL. *Consumer Reports* says, "Some studies have found that people with diets high in omega-3s—which are found in fatty fish such as salmon—may have a lower risk of dementia. But similar benefits are *not* linked to supplements. A 2012 review of data on thousands of older adults found that those who took omega-3 fatty acid supplements had no fewer dementia diagnoses or better scores on tests of short-term memory than those who took a placebo."[47] *Natural Medicines* writes, "Observational research has found conflicting associations between dietary fish and fish oil intake and cognitive function. Most clinical research shows that fish oil supplementation does NOT improve cognitive function in healthy elderly individuals, elderly patients with self-reported cognitive decline, or adults." For more information about fish oil, see the appendix.

GINKGO. Ginkgo is one of the most commonly used natural medicines in the elderly to boost cognitive function and improve symptoms of Alzheimer's disease and dementia. *Natural Medicines* says, "Although most evidence shows that ginkgo may improve symptoms of dementia, ginkgo does not appear to benefit age-related cognitive decline. Despite some conflicting evidence, most research shows that ginkgo does not improve memory or attention in elderly individuals. Don't recommend it." They add, "Furthermore, numerous case reports have documented serious bleeding events in patients taking ginkgo, especially when taken with aspirin, blood thinners, or antiplatelet drugs."

In December 2019, *Natural Medicines* warned, "Ginkgo products produced by lower-quality manufacturers are commonly adulterated with both rutin and quercetin. These chemicals both occur naturally in ginkgo, so adding them to ginkgo products makes the products much cheaper to produce while still appearing high quality to consumers and in some tests. Of the 35 analyzed ginkgo supplements, 33 contained low levels of ginkgo and/or high levels of rutin and quercetin. While products adulterated with rutin and quercetin shouldn't pose major safety concerns, there isn't evidence supporting their effectiveness for many of the common uses for ginkgo." They tell us doctors, "If your patients are interested in taking a ginkgo supplement, tell them to stick to products verified by a third party. . . . Also, remind patients that herbal combination products, particularly those manufactured overseas, are frequently tainted with drugs and heavy metals."

If you choose to try Ginkgo, based on quality, dosage, and value, ConsumerLab.com's "Top Pick" among the tested ginkgo extract supplements is *Life Extension Ginkgo Biloba.* ConsumerLab writes, "It provides the dose of ginkgo most commonly used in clinical trials (120 mg) and the correct concentrations of flavanol glycosides and terpene lactones, showed no sign of adulteration (based on tests for unhydrolyzed quercetin and rutin), and costs the least among the 'Approved' products to obtain 120 mg of ginkgo extract—just 9 cents per vegetarian capsule. To get the same amount of ginkgo extract from the other 'Approved' products would cost 2 to 30 times as much. Some of the more expensive products included other ingredients with some evidence of an effect on memory or cognition, but none of these formulas have been clinically proven to work, let alone been clinically tested." *Natural Medicines* lists no USP®-Verified ginkgo-only products, and Labdoor has tested no ginkgo products.

HUPERZINE A is isolated from Chinese club moss. *Natural Medicines* writes, "Several clinical trials evaluating huperzine A support its use for dementia. Taking huperzine A orally seems to improve memory, cognitive function, and behavioral function when taken for up to thirty-six weeks in patients with Alzheimer disease. Mood and activities of daily living also seem to improve with use of huperzine A in some of these patients." They add, "Preliminary clinical research suggests that taking huperzine A might also be beneficial for cognition in patients with senile or multi-infarct/vascular dementia" but conclude, "further research is needed in these patients."

ConsumerLab points out, "Some studies suggest huperzine A may enhance the effects of prescription drugs [for mild to moderate AD] donepezil (*Aricept®*) or tacrine (*Cognex®*), permitting lower doses of these drugs and fewer side effects from them." Also, ConsumerLab warns, "Be aware that supplements that list huperzine A may contain more or less huperzine A than claimed on the label, and/or potentially dangerous unlisted ingredients."

In fact, ConsumerLab "Approved" only three of six products they tested: *GNC Herbal Plus Standardized Huperzine A; Source Naturals® Huperzine A;* and *Swanson® Superior Herbs Maximum-Strength Huperzine A.* Regarding cost, ConsumerLab reports, "The cost of huperzine A ranged widely among the products. To obtain 100 mcg of huperzine A, the lowest cost was just 8 cents from *Source Naturals® Huperzine A*, followed by 17 cents from *Swanson® Superior Herbs Maximum-Strength Huperzine A*, and 76 cents from the GNC product. A similar amount of huperzine A from *Metagenics® Ceriva™* cost $1.39—seventeen times as much as from *Source Naturals®*." They add, "*Source Naturals®* was the only 'Approved' product which was vegetarian and gluten-free."

Another analysis from the Uniformed Services University and the National Center for Natural Products Research evaluated twenty-two products (tablets, capsules, and powders) listing huperzine A as an ingredient. These were all purchased online in the US. The researchers found that only two of the products contained within ten percent of the amount of huperzine A listed on their labels. Sixteen products (73 percent) contained ingredients not listed on the label, and nine products (41 percent) listed ingredients not meeting the regulations for being a dietary supplement ingredient, according to the FDA. One product labeled as "decaffeinated" contained caffeine. The researchers warned, "Some ingredients not on the label could be dangerous."[48] Labdoor has tested no huperzine A products, and *Natural Medicines* lists no USP®-"Verified" products (and, in fact, no product with a NMBER® rating above 7 out of 10).

SELENIUM. Cochrane concludes, "Selenium alone, taken for around five years, has no effect on the incidence of dementia."[49] *Natural Medicines* rates it as having "Insufficient Evidence" for preventing dementia. ConsumerLab points to a major placebo-controlled study among men in the US that found high-dose selenium and vitamin E did not reduce the risk of developing dementia over a thirteen-year period but was associated with a significant increase in hair loss and dermatitis.

VITAMIN D. *Natural Medicines* writes, "Population research has found that low vitamin D levels are associated with worse cognitive performance and cognitive decline compared to high vitamin D levels in healthy adults. However, the effect of vitamin D supplementation on cognitive function is unclear." They add, "Additional trials are needed to determine if dietary or supplemental vitamin D improves cognitive function." However, ConsumerLab concludes, "Supplementing with vitamin D may modestly improve cognition in older individuals with mild cognitive impairment who are vitamin D deficient, but it will not boost cognitive performance in adults who are not cognitively impaired."

ZINC and COPPER SUPPLEMENTATION. Cochrane advises, "Moderate-certainty evidence suggests that this has little or no effect on overall cognitive function, or the incidence of cognitive impairment, after five to ten years."[50] *Natural Medicines* rates zinc as having "Insufficient Evidence" for the treatment of AD or dementia, while copper was rated "Possibly Ineffective" for treating AD.

CITICOLINE, COCONUT OIL (MCTs or MEDIUM CHAIN TRI-GLYCERIDES), PHOSPHATIDYLSERINE, and RESVERATROL have been researched but the results are inconsistent. *Natural Medicines'* experts conclude that although each may be "promising, it is too early to recommend [them] for preventing age-related memory loss."

I hope you see the value of lifestyle habits over individual natural medicines for brain health. However, there are countless products that mix natural medicines and other ingredients; it almost seems there's a new one every week! Are any of them worth a hoot? We'll look at that in our next chapter, and then I'll include summary charts at the end of chapter 7.

7

Brain Health—Part 2

Combinations of Natural Medicines

An almost endless array of products is hyped for brain health. They include a wide variety of combinations of natural medicines, including B vitamins, antioxidant vitamins, dietary supplements, herbal products, and minerals. According to the experts at Cochrane, all studied products "have little or no effect on cognitive function." They add, "We did not find evidence that any vitamin or mineral supplementation strategy for cognitively healthy adults in mid or late life has a meaningful effect on cognitive decline or dementia . . . [even after up to] 8.5 years of taking them."[1] Here are some of the more popular brands. I think you'll detect a common theme.

BRAIN BRIGHT™ is a popular product that, according to the company website (which claims to be "Naturally Honest™"), is a brain-boosting supplement that "features 6 research-backed ingredients to help recharge a low-battery brain, supports mental focus and clarity, supports mental energy, supports a healthy mood, helps ease feelings of stress."[2]

ConsumerLab.com says it "contains several ingredients in doses which some small studies suggest may help to improve memory and cognition. However, there are no published clinical studies showing that these ingredients are safe or effective when taken together, as in the *Brain Bright*™

formula. Furthermore, the overall evidence for two of its main ingredients, ginkgo and *Rhodiola*, is currently considered insufficient for memory and cognition, and the evidence for the other ingredients is quite preliminary." The *Natural Medicines*™ NMBER® rating for *Brain Bright*™ is 5 out of 10. I never recommend products NMBER rated below 8.

NOVUSETIN® is a popular product containing the flavonoid antioxidant fisetin found in many fruits and vegetables. The maker of *Novusetin*® says it "promotes cognition and overall brain health."[3] *Natural Medicines* notes, "This product was formerly known as *Cognizin*. This is a 'branded ingredient,' meaning that it is an ingredient used in other companies' products. For example, this product might be just one component used in another company's product that contains multiple constituents. These branded products usually are not available for sale as stand-alone merchandise for consumers." ConsumerLab reports, "Results with fisetin in cells and animals are intriguing, but it is too early to know if fisetin is safe and effective for improving memory or any other condition in people at this time." *Natural Medicines*' NMBER rating for *Novusetin*® by *Cyvex Nutrition* and *Fisetin with Novusetin*® by *Doctor's Best* are both 5 out of 10.

NEURIVA is also growing in popularity. *Natural Medicines* says, "It contains coffee fruit extract, also known as *coffee cherry extract* or *green coffee*, and phosphatidylserine. While there is evidence that taking phosphatidylserine might improve age-related cognitive impairment and Alzheimer disease, evidence isn't good enough to recommend it for these conditions. And neither green coffee nor phosphatidylserine has been evaluated for improving general cognitive function." *Natural Medicines* NMBER rating for *Neuriva Original* and *Neuriva Plus* are both 6 out of 10.

PREVAGEN® is a trendy supplement that contains apoaequorin, a protein isolated from a specific jellyfish species, *Aequorea victoria*, as the active ingredient. The manufacturer has a huge advertising budget, and millions of people are being deceived. Every scientist I contacted or interviewed about *Prevagen*® said, "Don't waste your money!" Let me show you why I agree.

Natural Medicines writes, "*Prevagen*® was listed as the number one pharmacist recommended memory support supplement in the 2020 *Pharmacy*

Times survey." ConsumerLab says, "According to the company's website, people who use *Prevagen*® (Quincy Bioscience) can experience improved memory, a sharper mind, and clearer thinking." It must be a very profitable product as *Media Profile* reported Quincy spent just "under $100 million on advertising in digital, print, and national TV in the last year."[4]

Natural Medicines tells healthcare professionals, "While the marketing campaigns are convincing, most of the research on this ingredient is still preliminary, unpublished, and funded by the manufacturer. Until more research is available, don't recommend this product." *Natural Medicines'* NMBER rating is 6 out of 10 (I never recommend a product below 8). Although they say it is "Possibly Safe," they add that there is "Insufficient Evidence" to recommend it for cognitive function, memory, or age-related cognitive decline.

But there's more to the *Prevagen*® story than this. In 2013, "the FDA issued a warning letter, stating that Quincy was selling 'unapproved new drugs'—and not dietary supplements." This was "based on the unverified health claims on its website and Facebook page of 'miraculous' cures of memory loss, including from Alzheimer's and dementia." The FDA further alleged that "Quincy failed to report more than 1,000 'adverse events' among *Prevagen*® users, including some that required hospitalization."[5]

Fast forward to 2017, when *NBC News* reported, "The Federal Trade Commission and New York's attorney general [Eric Schneiderman] charged [the] makers of . . . *Prevagen*® are falsely advertising it as a memory booster."[6] Mr. Schneiderman said, "The marketing for *Prevagen*® is a clear-cut fraud, from the label on the bottle to the ads airing across the country."[7]

In 2018 *Science-Based Medicine* reported,

> Quincy's claims are rejected by the research community, which notes that any protein taken by mouth will be broken down into amino acids in the stomach and won't reach the brain in its original form.
>
> Quincy's claims "have no legitimate reality based on the real facts of science, nutrition, and memory," says David Mead, a molecular biologist and cofounder of Varigen Biosciences in Madison. "It's quackery. I can't think of anything better to say," says Baron Chanda, an associate professor in the UW-Madison Department of Neuroscience. "I second the 'quackery,'" says Chanda's neuroscience colleague, professor Edwin Chapman. "This is downright silly—no other word for it."

"The makers of *Prevagen®* are 'deceiving millions of aging Americans with claims that the supplement can treat age-related memory loss," said AARP® in a 2018 brief supporting the federal false advertising lawsuit. "The statements Quincy Bioscience makes to sell *Prevagen®*—that it treats memory loss—are unsubstantiated and misleading. . . . Supplement companies have keyed into the idea that older people are going to spend a ton of money on their products because they want to feel better. . . . We don't think they should get to prey on people's fears or claim their product offers some health benefit they cannot prove."[8]

Sarah Lenz Lock, executive director of the Global Council on Brain Health and senior vice president for policy at AARP®, added, "*Prevagen®* is popular because people are desperate for a cure for dementia-related diseases such as Alzheimer's. In the absence of a cure, companies offer supplements and make unfounded claims about their effectiveness. . . . Older people are clearly one of the biggest targets of the supplement industry."[9]

But as we were going to press, *Natural Medicines* reported, "Quincy Bioscience, the *Prevagen®* manufacturer, recently settled a nationwide class action lawsuit for making deceptive claims. Under the settlement agreement, Quincy must update product labeling, removing deceptive claims and adding appropriate disclaimers. They also must provide partial refunds to about three million consumers." One lawyer involved in the case wrote, "Each of those three million consumers opened his or her wallet in good faith and was sold a bottle of lies."[10]

"The settlement . . . is subject to court approval," *Daily Business Review* reported. "The ruling could provide a check on the competitive and lucrative field of consumer supplements. . . . The cost of this settlement may limit future product claims on other supplements that cross the line between puffery and actual violation of various consumer protection laws . . . [and] could be one of the largest consumer class settlements in the country . . . awarding tens of millions in damages."[11]

Natural Medicines advises health professionals, "If patients ask you about *Prevagen®*, tell them there's no convincing evidence that it works—and it's likely not worth the $40 [up to $100] for a monthly supply. Instead, recommend regular exercise, proper sleep, and a balanced diet to support cognitive health." I couldn't agree more.

QUALIA. *Natural Medicines* writes, "Other popular products on the market like *Qualia Mind™* [or *Qualia Focus™*] contain long lists of ingredients. While research supports some ingredients, there isn't enough data to know if they will offer any long-term benefits. . . . *Qualia Mind*™ in particular costs over $100 per bottle."

POMEGRANATE JUICE. Perhaps the best-known product is *POM Wonderful®*, which brags about its "tireless marketing efforts to let people know that we're THE Antioxidant Superpower, and we can help you get crazy healthy by drinking *POM Wonderful®*."[12] But dig a bit deeper into their website and you'll find they admit that the "early scientific findings on cognitive health and the impact of pomegranate juice on the human brain has not yet been adequately studied. Clinical research is needed to help establish causation, and further studies on larger populations are needed to confirm the long-term effect of pomegranate juice on memory and cognition."[13]

ConsumerLab recommends, "Until more is known, it seems generally safe to use pomegranate juice (other than potential allergic reactions), but its benefits remain largely unproven. The composition of pomegranate products on the market may vary significantly due to a lack of standards, and an optimal dosage has not been established."

OTHERS. On top of all this, in 2019, the FTC announced that multiple "brain boosting" supplements were promoted with "non-existent clinical studies." A 2019 ConsumerLab report explained, "The FTC announced the marketers of cognitive enhancement supplements *Geniux®*, *Xcel®*, *EVO®* (*Evodia*), and *Ion-Z®* have agreed to settle charges that they made false claims about the product, including fake research references and celebrity endorsements. The supplements were sold for $47 to $57 per bottle." *Natural Medicines* adds, "Furthermore, they can be very expensive."

A Waste of Money?

It's no wonder *Consumer Reports* concludes, "Our experts recommend avoiding branded 'memory boosting' blends."[14] Other groups are becoming increasingly vocal about the "money-wasting purchases" of many older people who are being deceived by the slick advertising of "brain supplements."

For example, *Consumer Reports* reviewed brain supplements, and Marvin M. Lipman, MD, *Consumer Reports'* chief medical adviser, concluded, "Don't be misled by hype. They are not only a waste of money, but some can also be harmful." Dr. Lipman added, "Supplements are also loosely regulated, and some may even contain undisclosed ingredients or prescription drugs. Many interact (sometimes dangerously) with medications—ginkgo biloba, for example, should never be paired with blood thinners, blood pressure meds, or SSRI antidepressants."[15]

AARP®'s GCBH bluntly warned that supplements to preserve or boost memory or cognition are not "worth the plastic they're bottled in."[16] Sarah Lenz Lock, the GCBH executive director, said, "Supplements for brain health appear to be a huge waste of money for the 25 percent of adults over 50 who take them."[17] AARP® found older adults spend more than $93 million a month on just six different "brain health" supplements. "These people taking these pills are spending between $20 and $60 a month and flushing dollars down the toilet that could be better spent on things that actually improve their brain health," Lock said.[18]

Ronald C. Petersen, MD, director of Mayo Clinic's Alzheimer's Disease Research Center and a member of the GCBH Governance Committee, said, "Given the lack of government regulation before their products hit the market, supplement or 'nutraceutical' makers have little incentive to provide scientific studies to back up any claims they may make." He added, "They can only lose market share by doing so."[19]

The GCBH report did mention one significant exception in cautioning against supplements for brain health: "For individuals diagnosed as being deficient in vitamin B12 [cobalamin] or [vitamin] B9 [folic acid], also known as *folate*, supplements may be helpful for brain health. [Vitamin] B12 deficiency, for example, has been associated with cognitive function problems, including dementia."[20]

Product Impurity

"Beyond the risk of wasting your money on something that won't make you one wit sharper," wrote Kathleen Fifield, "the [GCBH] report also warns against 'vague or exaggerated claims about brain health' for some supplements as well as potential product impurities and inaccurate ingredient labels."[21]

Natural Medicines adds, "Some products can also pose safety risks, interact with drugs, and many have been shown to contain unlisted ingredients like phenibut." Phenibut, or beta-phenyl-gamma-aminobutyric acid, is rated as "Possibly Unsafe" by *Natural Medicines*, adding, "Short-term use of phenibut has been associated with delirium, diminished consciousness, reduced respirations, and sedation. Phenibut is also addictive [and] has been associated with . . . withdrawal symptoms including aggression, anxiety, agitation, hallucinations, insomnia, and seizure."

Harvard Medical School's Pieter A. Cohen, MD, and his team have found another example of product contamination. In a 2019 report in *JAMA Internal Medicine*, they reported that a drug rejected by the FDA was found in five brands of brain-boosting supplements.[22] The drug, piracetam, has been approved in the EU for the treatment of cognitive impairment in dementia but has been rejected by the FDA as a dietary supplement in the US after a major review of twenty-four studies involving eleven thousand patients found it had little impact on cognition.[23] While the typical dose of the drug in Europe is between 2,400 mg and 4,800 mg, if the supplements sold in the US are "taken as labeled, a user could ingest more than 11,000 mg daily."[24] Common adverse effects of piracetam at recommended doses include anxiety, insomnia, agitation, depression, drowsiness, and weight gain.[25] Dr. Cohen warns, "This drug is just the tip of the iceberg of how companies introduce a variety of unapproved drugs in 'cognitive enhancement' supplements."[26]

In 2020, Cohen and colleagues identified and purchased ten so-called "nootropic" or "cognitive enhancer" supplements that they were suspicious contained omberacetam (Noopept), a piracetam analog used in Russia to treat traumatic brain injury, mood disorders, cerebral vascular disease, and other indications but not approved in the US. His findings were very concerning. He says, "Not only did we detect five unapproved drugs in these products, we also detected several drugs that were not mentioned on the labels, and we found doses of unapproved drugs that were as much as four times higher than what would be considered a typical dose."[27]

The Bottom Line: Your Best Options

Joshua Sharfstein, MD, of Johns Hopkins Bloomberg School of Public Health and a former FDA deputy commissioner, told *MedPage Today* that it is "nearly impossible for the FDA to keep these [drugs and supplements] off the market with current laws."[28] Dr. Cohen added that "until laws governing supplements are reformed, clinicians should advise patients that supplements marketed as cognitive enhancers may contain prohibited drugs."[29] Jacob Hall, MD, added, "Although more research is always needed, no supplements have been proven to be effective in treating or preventing cognitive decline. Except in specific medical conditions, they're a waste of money and, in some cases, potentially dangerous."[30]

In its 2018 review, *Consumer Reports* agreed, concluding, "According to a review of studies published . . . there's virtually no good evidence that such products can prevent or delay memory lapses, mild cognitive impairment, or dementia in older adults. In fact, says Pieter Cohen, MD, . . . some may do more harm than good."[31]

Based on all of this, the 2018 American Academy of Neurology (AAN) practice guideline recommended that "patients and families be counseled that there are currently no dietary modalities (vitamin or mineral supplementation) effective in slowing symptomatic cognitive impairment."[32]

Finally, a 2020 review concluded, "Vitamin and mineral supplementation has little to no beneficial effect on preserving cognitive functioning or preventing dementia in cognitively healthy adults 40 years or older."[33]

So what options do people have to prevent or treat early dementia? The World Health Organization (WHO) has created guidelines that include the following:

- *Lifestyle habits.* Quit smoking, limit alcohol consumption, and maintain a healthy weight.
- *Dietary habits.* The Mediterranean diet, which emphasizes an olive oil, fish, nut, whole grain, fruit, and vegetable intake is linked to a 46 percent reduced risk for dementia or Alzheimer's disease, but strict adherence is necessary to get these benefits. That might not be realistic for all patients, so other diet options including the DASH (Dietary Approaches to Stop Hypertension) diet can be recommended as well.

- *Supplements.* The WHO recommends against their use. Specifically, the guidelines recommend against B and E vitamins, polyunsaturated fatty acids such as fish oil, and multivitamins.

Commenting on the WHO report, *Natural Medicines* tells health professionals, "These recommendations may be important to highlight, as your patients may have heard unsupported claims that some of these supplements are beneficial. For instance, fish oil is often touted as being a 'brainfood,' but the evidence in relation to dementia doesn't support this claim. Similarly, the use of multivitamins as a strategy for staying healthy is common, but strong evidence of benefit for dementia is lacking."

In addition to the above, instead of "wasting your money on brain supplements," *Consumer Report*'s Dr. Marvin Lipman suggests the following:[34]

- *Do a brain workout.* Enhancing reasoning and memory abilities—learning a new language, for instance—might help delay or slow decline. A ten-year trial found that such training (though not computerized "brain games") can help increase cognitive processing speed and sharpen reasoning skills.
- *Exercise your body.* In 2011, one study estimated that one million cases of Alzheimer's disease in the US were due to sedentary lifestyle. Several studies have found that physical activity—walking, weightlifting, yoga, or tai chi, for example—may delay or slow cognitive decline but not prevent it.
- *Manage blood pressure.* Lowering blood pressure dramatically reduces the risk of heart disease and stroke, which are risk factors for memory loss.

To Dr. Lipman's list, I would add the Mediterranean diet. According to a 2020 study,[35] "Yet more bragging rights are in for the Mediterranean diet, long considered to be one of the healthiest in the world. The study found . . . that eating the Mediterranean diet for just one year altered . . . elderly people in ways that improved brain function and would aid in longevity. . . . The diet can inhibit production of inflammatory chemicals that can lead to loss of cognitive function and prevent the development of chronic diseases such as diabetes, cancer and atherosclerosis."[36]

A CNN report added, "Discovering that the Mediterranean diet could affect the [elderly] in a positive way isn't really surprising; the diet already has a stuffed shelf of scientific trophies. It's won gold medals in reducing the risk for diabetes, high cholesterol, dementia, memory loss, depression and breast cancer. Meals from the sunny Mediterranean region have also been linked to stronger bones, a healthier heart and longer life. Oh, and weight loss, too."[37]

Atlanta dietitian Rahaf Al Bochi, RDN, LD, told CNN, "It's more than a diet, it's a lifestyle," adding, "It also encourages eating with friends and family, socializing over meals, mindfully eating your favorite foods, as well as mindful movement and exercise."[38]

Also, see my discussion about the MIND diet in chapter 6, "Brain Health —Part 1."

Space constraints prevent me from discussing with you the myriad studies on treating dementia or Alzheimer's disease with natural medicines, so I'll just share *Natural Medicines*' conclusions in the chart below. Also, I've included many commonly used natural medicines that aren't discussed in the chapter. More detailed information is available from ConsumerLab .com and *Natural Medicines*.

Natural Interventions and Medications to Prevent or Delay Age-Related Memory Loss or Cognitive Impairment

Effective \ Safe	Likely Safe	Possibly Safe
Effective	★★★★★ • Avoid sedentary activity • Avoid tobacco products • Folic acid (vitamin B9) to treat memory loss associated with folate deficiency • Mediterranean diet • MIND diet • Nutrient-dense foods (fruits, vegetables, lean protein, heart-healthy fats) • Regular exercise • Restful sleep • Vitamin B12 (cobalamin) to treat memory loss associated with B12 deficiency	★★★

Safe / Effective	Likely Safe	Possibly Safe
Likely Effective	★★★★ • Manage medical problems such as hypertension, diabetes, depression, and obstructive sleep apnea • Mental stimulation, cognitive-stimulating activities • Reduce or manage stress	★★
Possibly Effective	★★★ • Acetyl-L-carnitine • Alcohol (beer/wine) in moderation • Avoid social isolation • Caffeine (<400 mg/day) • Connect socially • Phosphatidylserine • Personal prayer, meditation, positive spirituality • Religious involvement	★ • Citicoline • Huperzine A

Insufficient evidence for safety or effectiveness AND/OR evidence for lack of safety or effectiveness	☹
	• A wide variety of combinations of various natural medicines (complex supplements):
	  • Brain Bright
	  • EVO
	  • Fisetin
	  • Geniux
	  • Ion-Z
	  • Neuriva
	  • Novusetin
	• Bacopa monnieri
	• Beta-carotene
	• B vitamins
	• Carnosine
	• Choline
	• Coconut oil
	• Fish oil
	• Folic acid (vitamin B9)
	• Ginkgo
		• Lecithin
		• L-Serine
		• MCTs
		• Mineral supplements
		• Noopept
		• Nootropics
		• Panax ginseng
		• Phenibut
		• Pomegranate juice
		• POM Wonderful
		• PQQ (Pyrroloquinoline quinone)
		• Prevagen
		• Qualia
		• Resveratrol
		• Rhodiola rosea
		• Vitamin B6 (pyridoxine)
		• Vitamin B12 (cobalamin)
		• Vitamin D

Natural Interventions and Medications to Prevent or Delay Dementia or Alzheimer's Disease

Effective / Safe	Likely Safe	Possibly Safe
Effective	★★★★★ • Avoid sedentary activity as much as possible • Avoid tobacco products • Folic acid (vitamin B9) to treat memory loss associated with folate deficiency • Mediterranean diet • MIND diet • Nutrient-dense foods (fruits, vegetables, lean protein, heart-healthy fats) • Regular exercise • Restful sleep • Vitamin B12 (cobalamin) to treat memory loss associated with B12 deficiency	★★
Likely Effective	★★★★ • Manage medical problems such as hypertension, diabetes, depression, and obstructive sleep apnea • Mental stimulation, cognitive-stimulating activities • Reduce or manage stress	★★
Possibly Effective	★★★ • Acetyl-L-carnitine • Ginkgo • Ginkgo leaf • Vitamin E (treating AD) • Wine (in moderation)	★ • Huperzine A • Phosphatidylserine • Vinpocetine

Insufficient evidence for safety or effectiveness AND/OR evidence for lack of safety or effectiveness	

 • A wide variety of combinations of various natural medicines (complex supplements):
   • Brain Bright
   • EVO
   • Fisetin
   • Geniux
   • Ion-Z
   • Neuriva
   • Novusetin
 • Beer (in moderation)
 • Beta-carotene
 • Butea superba
 • B vitamins
 • Caprylic acid
 • Choline
 • Coconut oil
	• DMAE
	 • Evening primrose oil
	 • Fish oil
	 • Folic acid (vitamin B9)
	 • Lecithin
	 • L-serine
	 • MCTs
	 • Mineral supplements
	 • Niacin (vitamin B3)
	 • Noopept
	 • Nootropics
	 • Turmeric
	 • Vitamin B6 (pyridoxine)
	 • Vitamin B9 (folic acid)
	 • Vitamin B12 (cobalamin)
	 • Vitamin C
	 • Vitamin E (preventing AD)

The recommendations in the charts are based almost entirely on the "Safety and Effectiveness Ratings" contained in *Natural Medicines™* and explained in chapter 4 of this book. They assume the use of high-quality, uncontaminated products and the use of typical doses. Keep in mind that some products are never appropriate for some patients due to concomitant disease states, potential drug interactions, or other clinical factors. Details are available at *Natural Medicines™*.

8

Cholesterol and Dyslipidemia

*L*ipid is another word for *fat*, and cholesterol is one of many lipids in our bodies. We need lipids to build healthy cells, but high levels of lipids in the bloodstream can build up in the walls of our arteries. Over the years or even decades, these deposits grow and can reduce blood flow. Even worse, these deposits can suddenly burst, causing a blood clot to form that can cause a heart attack or stroke.

According to the CDC, ninety-five million US adults age twenty or older have elevated blood cholesterol levels (> 200 mg/dL). Nearly twenty-nine million adult Americans have very high total cholesterol levels (> 240 mg/dL). The danger is that those with raised cholesterol levels have about twice the risk of developing cardiovascular disease, including heart attacks and strokes, as people with normal levels. Furthermore, slightly less than half of the adults who could benefit from cholesterol medicine are taking it.[1]

However, the story is far more complicated than just high cholesterol. *Dyslipidemia* is the term for when a person has an abnormal amount of lipids in their bloodstream. It includes high levels of the dangerous low-density lipoprotein (LDL), also called *bad* or *lethal* cholesterol, or high levels of potentially harmful triglycerides (TG) called *hypertriglyceridemia*. Also, it can include abnormally low levels of high-density lipoprotein (HDL), also called *good* or *healthy* cholesterol. I teach my patients that the *H* in HDL stands for "healthy cholesterol," while the *L* in LDL stands for "lethal cholesterol." In general, the higher the HDL and the lower the LDL and TG, the better.

A blood test (measuring total cholesterol, LDL cholesterol, HDL cholesterol, and triglycerides) is the easiest and most economical way to detect abnormalities in your blood lipids. *Natural Medicines™* advises, "Heart-healthy lifestyle choices such as healthy diet and regular exercise are recommended to *all* patients with dyslipidemia. Those with a high enough risk may also qualify for drug therapy involving a statin." But drug therapy should typically be used only if lifestyle changes do not work.

The American Heart Association (AHA) says, "In all individuals, emphasize a heart-healthy lifestyle across the life course. A healthy lifestyle reduces atherosclerotic cardiovascular disease (ASCVD) risk at all ages. In younger individuals, healthy lifestyle can reduce development of risk factors and is the foundation of ASCVD risk reduction. In young adults 20 to 39 years of age, an assessment of lifetime risk facilitates the clinician-patient risk discussion and emphasizes intensive lifestyle efforts." AHA adds, "In all age groups, lifestyle therapy is the primary intervention. When lifestyle interventions alone are not enough to lower LDL, statins generally provide the most effective lipid-lowering treatment."[2]

Diets—Which Ones Are Best?

Several nutritional approaches benefit both dyslipidemia and hypertension, resulting in significant reductions in the risk of cardiovascular disease, including heart attacks, heart failure, and stroke. Which method is the best? Each year, the editors of *US News and World Reports* convene "a panel of food and health experts to rank 40 diets on a variety of measures."[3] In their 2020 ratings for the best "Heart-Healthy Diets," the Ornish diet was first, followed by the Mediterranean and DASH diets.[4]

ORNISH DIET. Most of my patients have not heard of the Ornish diet. *US News* says, "The Ornish Diet was created in 1977 by Dr. Dean Ornish—a clinical professor of medicine at the University of California, San Francisco . . . to help people 'feel better, live longer, lose weight and gain health.' The plan is low in fat, refined carbohydrates, and animal protein, which Ornish says makes it ideal. But it's not just a diet: his strategy also emphasizes exercise, stress management, and relationships." *US News* says the pros are that it's "solid nutritionally" and "your heart will love you." The cons are that "staying the course could be tough if you're aiming to reverse heart disease" and it's "not exactly cheap."[5]

MEDITERRANEAN DIET. Number two in heart-healthy diets is the Mediterranean diet. *US News* says, "It's generally accepted that the folks in countries bordering the Mediterranean Sea live longer and suffer less than most Americans from cancer and cardiovascular ailments. The not-so-surprising secret is an active lifestyle, weight control, and a diet low in red meat, sugar and saturated fat and high in produce, nuts and other healthful foods. The Mediterranean Diet may offer a host of health benefits, including weight loss, heart and brain health, cancer prevention, and diabetes prevention and control. By following the Mediterranean Diet, you could also keep that weight off while avoiding chronic disease."[6] The pros are that it is "nutritionally sound" and "diverse [in] foods and flavors," while the cons are that it is "lots of grunt work" and "moderately pricey."[7]

US News adds, "There isn't 'a' Mediterranean diet. Greeks eat differently from Italians, who eat differently from the French and Spanish. But they share many of the same principles."[8] Working with the Harvard School of Public Health, Oldways, a nonprofit food think tank in Boston, developed a consumer-friendly Mediterranean diet pyramid that offers guidelines on how to fill your plate—and maybe wine glass—the Mediterranean way.[9]

DASH DIET. The third-place heart-healthy diet is the DASH diet. *US News* reports it "is promoted by the National Heart, Lung, and Blood Institute" and "emphasizes the foods you've always been told to eat (fruits, veggies, whole grains, lean protein, and low-fat dairy), which are high in blood pressure-deflating nutrients like potassium, calcium, protein and fiber. DASH also discourages foods that are high in saturated fat, such as fatty meats, full-fat dairy foods, and tropical oils, as well as sugar-sweetened beverages and sweets. Following DASH also means capping sodium at 2,300 milligrams a day, which followers will eventually lower to about 1,500 milligrams." The DASH diet is balanced and can be followed long term, which is a key reason nutrition experts rank it as *US News'* tied for second-best "Overall Diet," with an overall score of 4.1 out of 5, just behind the Mediterranean diet. The pros are that it is "nutritionally sound" and "heart healthy," while the cons are that it is "lots of grunt work" and "somewhat pricey."[10]

PLANT-BASED DIETS. In the "Best Plant-Based Diet" category, the experts chose, in this order, the Mediterranean diet, the Flexitarian diet, and the Nordic diet. In "The Easiest Diet to Follow," the Mediterranean diet was once again tops followed by a second-place tie between the Flexitarian diet and the DASH diet. The "Best Weight-Loss Diet" was Weight Watchers, followed by the Vegan diet.[11]

BEST DIETS OVERALL. In the "Best Diets Overall," "The Best Diets for Healthy Eating," and "The Best Diets for Diabetes," the Mediterranean diet came in first place, followed by a second-place tie between the DASH diet and the Flexitarian diet. Taken together, it seems to me these three are the best to consider—with the Mediterranean diet nosing slightly ahead of the others.

Natural Medicines rates the Mediterranean diet as "Likely Safe" and "Possibly Effective" for cardiovascular disease (CVD), cognitive function, dementia, and diabetes; "Possibly Ineffective" for hypertension; and "Insufficient Evidence" for cancer. As for the DASH diet, *Natural Medicines* rates it "Likely Safe" and "Likely Effective" for hypertension; "Possibly Effective" for CVD, hyperlipidemia, and weight loss; and "Insufficient Evidence" for diabetes or overall mortality.

FLEXITARIAN DIET. About the Flexitarian diet, *US News* says, "Flexitarian is a marriage of two words: *flexible* and *vegetarian*. The term was coined more than a decade ago . . . in [a] 2009 book [*sic*, it was published in 2008[12]] . . . [that] says you don't have to eliminate meat completely to reap the health benefits associated with vegetarianism—you can be a vegetarian most of the time, but still chow down on a burger or steak when the urge hits. By eating more plants and less meat, it's suggested that adherents to the diet will not only lose weight but can improve their overall health, lowering their rate of heart disease, diabetes and cancer, and live longer as a result."[13]

The pros are that the Flexitarian diet is "flexible" with "lots of (tasty) recipes," and the cons are the "emphasis on home cooking" and it "might be tough if you don't like fruits and veggies"[14]—although I would consider cooking at home to be a great thing. *Natural Medicines* rates the "semi-vegetarian" Flexitarian diet as well as other vegetarian diets as "Likely Safe" and "Possibly Effective" for diabetes, hypertension, and obesity and "Insufficient Evidence" for cancer, CVD, hypercholesterolemia, and overall mortality.

Overall, *US News* rates the Mediterranean diet 4.2 out of 5, while giving the DASH and Flexitarian diets a 4.1 out of 5 rating. The Mediterranean rates #1 in the categories "Best Diets Overall," "Best Plant-Based Diets," "Best Diabetes Diets," and "Easiest Diets to Follow," while falling to #2 in "Best Heart-Healthy Diets" (after Ornish and ahead of DASH).[15]

Therefore, the Mediterranean diet is my number-one recommendation—and is also recommended or very highly rated by the AHA,[16] the American Society for Nutrition,[17] the Cleveland Clinic,[18] *Consumer Reports*,[19] the European Food Information Council,[20] Johns Hopkins,[21] the Harvard School of Public Health,[22] Mayo Clinic,[23] *Today's Dietitian* (the trade publication for registered dietitians and other nutrition professionals),[24] Tufts University,[25] the Women's Heart Foundation,[26] the WHO,[27] the USDA,[28] and many other universities as well as national and international medical and health groups.

Exercise versus "Sitting Disease"

The editors of *Reader's Digest* tell us, "What is arguably the most common health problem in America today [is] *sitting disease*."[29] In fact, a 2020 study from the CDC concluded more than "one in seven adults across all US states and territories are physically inactive." They define physical inactivity "as doing no leisure-time physical activities in the past month—such as running, walking for exercise, or gardening." Across the US, "southern states had the highest rate of inactivity (28 percent), followed by the Northeast (26 percent), Midwest (25 percent), and the West (21 percent)."[30]

Researchers from the University of Cambridge reported sitting too much is twice as likely to lead to premature death as being obese![31] Cleveland Clinic investigators reported a clear connection between exercise and longer, healthier life. Cleveland Clinic cardiologist and study author Wael A. Jaber, MD, told CNN, "Being unfit . . . had a worse prognosis, as far as death, than being hypertensive, being diabetic, or being a current smoker." He added, "We've never seen something as pronounced as this." He concluded that lack of exercise "should be treated as a disease that has a prescription, which is called *exercise*."[32] Regular exercise increases longevity, reduces fatigue and disability, reduces the risk of heart disease, and improves mental health.

Statins

When diet and exercise fail to control dyslipidemia, by far the most effective, safe, and economical treatment for abnormal lipids is a class of prescription drugs called *statins* or *HMG-CoA reductase inhibitors*. They block the production of cholesterol. The experts at *Natural Medicines* conclude, "Statins can lower LDL cholesterol by up to 55 percent. Plus, they can boost HDL cholesterol levels by 5 to 15 percent. Patients who take a statin have a significantly reduced risk of adverse cardiovascular outcomes such as heart attack and stroke." The AHA adds, "Research shows statins may lower heart attack risk by at least 25 percent and may also help patients with heart disease avoid cardiac procedures such as coronary stents."[33]

Unlike natural medicines, statins are pharmaceutical-grade products. Furthermore, they can be far, far less expensive than over-the-counter products, and almost all insurance plans cover them. But, even so, pharmacy coupons or cash prices may be even lower. For example, the lowest GoodRx .com (my favorite website for comparative drug prices) cost for several commonly prescribed and very effective statins where I live is below $20 for a three-month supply, and in the case of atorvastatin (generic *Lipitor®*), for less than $7 for a three-month supply—less than 7 cents a day!

Are there potential side effects? Absolutely! Remember what I told you earlier? "If a medication (even a natural medication) does not have side effects, then it will have *no* effects!" However, as the AHA advises, "The benefits of the cholesterol-lowering medicines called *statins* far outweigh any risk of side effects, according to a new analysis of decades of scientific research. In fact, side effects of statins are rare."[34] Nevertheless, whether to take a statin is a surprisingly complicated question and beyond the scope of this book. CNN has an excellent article on the topic.[35]

Plant Sterols/Stanols

Natural Medicines instructs health professionals, "For patients who want to incorporate a natural approach into their treatment, there are several viable options including plant sterols/stanols." ConsumerLab.com says, "Plant-based sterols and stanols . . . are produced in the refinement of vegetable oils. . . . The FDA permits sterol-containing products to claim that they help reduce the risk of heart disease when used with a diet low in saturated fat and cholesterol. For a manufacturer to make this claim, their product must provide a total of 800 mg of free sterols (1.3 grams of sterol esters) divided into at least two servings per day and taken with meals."

ConsumerLab adds, "It should be noted that while sterols and stanols can lower cholesterol, no study has shown a direct reduction in the risk of cardiovascular disease." *Natural Medicines* agrees, concluding, "Keep in mind that these products have only been shown to reduce cholesterol, a risk factor for heart disease. They have not been shown to reduce the risk of cardiovascular outcomes, such as heart attack."

Nevertheless, as *Natural Medicines* points out, "Plant sterols and stanols are now considered mainstream. Plant sterols are in *Promise*® *Activ Spread*, *Smart Balance*® *Buttery Spread*, *Minute Maid*® *Premium Heart Wise* orange juice, and many other products. Stanols are in *Benecol*® spreads and others."

For those choosing to take a sterol/stanol supplement, among ConsumerLab's "Approved" products is their "Top Pick": *Nature Made*® *Cholest-Off*® *Plus*. ConsumerLab says, "It provides the right ingredients at the best price and even has a clinical study to support its efficacy. Each two-softgel dose claims to provide 900 mg of a combination of sterols and stanols." ConsumerLab adds, "Our tests showed that it did (actually, it contained 96.5 percent of this, but this is within an acceptable range) and the vast majority of this was from sterols. . . . *CholestOff*® *Plus* is also in the ester form, which may be more effective than the free form, and it is in softgel form, which may be more effective than a tablet."

In addition, "*CholestOff*® *Plus* was, by far, the least expensive source of sterols/stanols, at just sixteen cents per 900 mg. The cost to obtain the same amount of sterols/stanols from other products ranged from forty-seven to seventy-four cents."

However, *Natural Medicines* warns that sterols, which are absorbed, could theoretically worsen cardiovascular outcomes. They advise, "Until more is known, some experts recommend only using plant stanol products (e.g., *Benecol®*, others), which are not absorbed, and avoid plant sterol products." The NMBER® ratings for *Benecol® Smart Chews* and *Benecol® Softgels* (McNeil Consumer Healthcare) are 9 out of 10; however, the *Benecol®* spreads (*Buttery, Light, Olive,* and *Soft Cheese*) are only rated 5 out of 10.

My recommendation is that if you're comfortable trying a sterol, *CholestOff® Plus* is the way to go. If not, then the *Benecol® Smart Chews* or *Softgels* may be for you.

High Fiber Foods for Dyslipidemia

Natural Medicines also recommends high-fiber foods, such as blond psyllium and whole grains. They explain, "Fibrous foods can also help lower cholesterol. The FDA permits health claims for some whole grain foods. Foods that contain at least fifty-one percent whole grains (whole wheat, whole oats, dried corn, barley) may claim to reduce the risk of heart disease. It's the fiber in whole grains that seems to reduce heart disease. The FDA also allows health claims for blond psyllium and oat bran due to their soluble fiber content."

"Blond psyllium is among the most studied sources of fiber," writes *Natural Medicines*. "Like other fibers, blond psyllium can decrease cholesterol by absorbing dietary fats in the GI tract, preventing systemic absorption, and increasing cholesterol elimination in fecal bile acids. Patients who consume 10 to 12 grams of blond psyllium per day can decrease total cholesterol by 3 to 14 percent, LDL cholesterol by 5 to 11 percent. . . . Blond psyllium seems to be most effective at lowering cholesterol when taken with food at mealtime. But blond psyllium doesn't seem to work when taken in doses of 6 grams daily or less."

For those not wanting to increase fiber in their diet, *Natural Medicines* lists over two hundred products in powder or capsules containing blond psyllium that are NMBER rated 9 out of 10. The powders come as "tasteless" or flavored and can often be mixed into food, juice, water, coffee, or tea. Labdoor is also planning to review fiber products.

Another source of fiber that has been shown to lower cholesterol are whole grains, particularly oats. *Natural Medicines* advises, "Clinical research shows that consuming 56 to 150 grams of whole oat products, such as oatmeal and oat bran . . . can significantly lower total cholesterol and LDL cholesterol . . . by about 4 to 14 mg/dL." They add, "Whole oat products might be more effective in lowering LDL cholesterol and total cholesterol," and tell us doctors to "explain to patients that the extent of cholesterol lowering that occurs while taking fiber is highly variable. It all depends on how much is consumed and the other contents of the diet. A person who consumes a high amount of fiber along with a low-fat diet will likely have the greatest reduction in cholesterol." I would say "A person who consumes a high amount of fiber along with a healthy-fat diet combined with regular exercise will have even greater reductions in bad cholesterol, weight, BMI, and blood sugar while increasing their good cholesterol."

ConsumerLab says, "Although oats don't naturally contain gluten, oat cereals may become cross-contaminated with gluten from wheat products during processing, a potential concern for some people." ConsumerLab tested products against the FDA standard for "gluten-free," as well as its own, more stringent "ultra-gluten-free" standard. If you like an oat cereal in the morning like I do, here are ConsumerLab's "Top Picks" based on product quality and cost per serving (forty grams of dry cereal):

- Steel-Cut ("Irish") Oats:
  - Regular: *Bob's Red Mill® Steel Cut Oats* (15 cents)
  - Quick Cook: *Trader Joe's® Quick Cook Steel Cut Oats* (15 cents)
- Rolled Oats:
  - Regular: *Quaker® Oats Old Fashioned* (17 cents)—it was also low in gluten (11 ppm [parts per million]), although lowest in gluten was *Trader Joe's® Rolled Oats* (18 cents).
  - Quick Cook: *365 Organic Quick Oats* (Whole Foods® Market) (23 cents)—it was also very low in gluten (6.6 ppm), although lowest in gluten was *Bob's Red Mill® Quick Cooking Oats* (31 cents) as it had less than 5 ppm, meeting not only its gluten-free claim but also ConsumerLab's more stringent ultra-gluten-free requirement.

- Instant Oats:
  - *Quaker® Instant Oatmeal Original* (42 cents)—It is more expensive than many other products but comes in a convenient packet and was very low in gluten (none detected above 5 ppm), making it ultra-gluten-free—although gluten-free is not claimed.

The Academy of Nutrition and Dietetics (AND) says, "Dietary fiber contributes to health and wellness in a number of ways:

1. It aids in providing fullness after meals, which helps promote a healthy weight.
2. Adequate fiber intake can help to lower cholesterol.
3. It helps prevent constipation and diverticulosis.
4. Adequate fiber from food helps keep glucose within a healthy range."[36]

AND cautions, "Many Americans fall far short of the recommended daily amount in their diets. Women should aim for 25 grams of fiber per day, while men should target 38 grams, or 14 grams for every 1,000 calories." They add, "Fiber is found in plant foods. Eating the skin or peel of fruits and vegetables provides a greater dose of fiber, which is found naturally in these sources. Fiber also is found in beans and lentils, whole grains, nuts and seeds. Typically, the more refined or processed a food is, the lower its fiber content. For example, one medium apple with the peel contains 4.4 grams of fiber, while ½ cup of applesauce contains 1.4 grams, and 4 ounces of apple juice contains no fiber."[37]

When it comes to fiber-rich breakfast cereals, *Consumer Reports* says they "have made progress on the road to tastiness." In tests they performed fourteen years ago, their lab reported that most high-fiber cereals "tasted more like straw than grain." But in subsequent tests of twenty-six cereals, most with at least 6 grams of fiber, "more than two-thirds tasted very good or better."[38] You just want to find a brand that's high in protein, whole grains, and fiber, with zero added sugar and zero sodium. Add fruit, a few nuts, and milk or yogurt, and you cover four bases at once: fruit, protein, a complex carbohydrate, and dairy.

EPA and DHA (Fish Oil) for Hypertriglyceridemia

Natural Medicines' experts advise physicians, "Fish oil is appropriate for patients with hypertriglyceridemia. Save krill oil for patients who can't tolerate fish oil. Don't recommend fish oil for hypercholesterolemic patients with normal triglyceride levels, as fish oil may increase LDL cholesterol levels."

Eicosapentaenoic acid (EPA, which is a long-chain polyunsaturated fatty acid [PUFA] derived from marine mammals and oily fish) is available as a natural medicine. However, it's also available by prescription. *Vascepa®* has been approved, along with diet modification, to reduce TG levels in adults with severe (≥ 500 mg/dL) high triglycerides (called *hypertriglyceridemia*). In December 2019 this approval was extended to include it in addition to statins to reduce the risk of cardiovascular events among adults with elevated TGs (≥ 150 mg/dL) who also have either established cardiovascular disease or diabetes and two or more additional risk factors for cardiovascular disease.

ConsumerLab writes, "Vascepa®, which has been shown to reduce the risk of cardiovascular disease in people with elevated levels of triglycerides, provides 960 mg of EPA per capsule, and two of these capsules are taken twice daily with meals. The cash price for each capsule is about $2.50, or $10 per day (pricing can vary, or an annual cost of approximately $3,000). InMay 2020, the FDA approved a generic competitor to Vascepa®, but in late 2020, its launch had not been announced, apparently due to ongoing patent dispute."

As discussed in ConsumerLab's *Review of Fish Oil Supplements*, "highly concentrated fish oil supplements can provide about the same amount of EPA with little DHA, like Vascepa®, but for as little as 30 percent the cost of Vascepa®." ConsumerLab also says, "Fish oil in softgels is generally the least expensive way to get good-quality EPA and DHA." Under its "Best Picks," ConsumerLab recommends:

GNC® *Triple Strength EPA* [which] can provide about the same amount of EPA (along with a bit more DHA) as Vascepa® at less than one-third the cost. Both appear to be ethyl esters. One difference between them, however, is that the GNC product is enteric coated, delaying its release of oils until after it passes through the stomach. While this may reduce "fishy burps," it's not clear how this may affect absorption. It's possible that earlier release of the oils in the gut could allow their earlier mixing and better stimulate the bile production needed for absorption of the oils in the small intestine. If that is of concern, one could potentially bite open the GNC softgel, negating the effect of the enteric coating.

Another option suggested by ConsumerLab to get the recommended amount of EPA (about 3,840 mg per day in divided doses) at an even lower cost is to purchase a fish oil product that is not as highly concentrated. However, these products "will likely include significant amounts of other omega-3 fatty acids . . . making the dose larger, i.e. more softgels, capsules, or liquid."

ConsumerLab also warns, "While EPA/DHA combinations, as found in the prescription fish oil Lovaza® and many supplements, can lower triglycerides, they have not, to date, been shown to lower the risk of cardiovascular disease like Vascepa®." They add, "A generic version of Lovaza is also available at lower cost. It is sold by Teva Pharmaceuticals as one-gram capsules of 'omega-3-acid ethyl esters' and was approved by the FDA as providing approximately the same amounts of EPA and DHA in the same chemical form as Lovaza."

As for its "Top Pick," ConsumerLab writes, "If cost is more of an issue than the size and number of pills you take, our 'Top Pick' is *Kirkland Signature™* [Costco®] *Fish Oil 1000 mg*, which provides 250 mg of EPA plus DHA as moderately concentrated fish oil in the 'triglyceride' form per softgel. The cost is just 3 cents per softgel, making it the most economical product at 1 cent per 100 mg of EPA and DHA. In addition, although not stated on the label, its omega-3s appear to be in the triglyceride form so that you're likely to get the best absorption."

ConsumerLab adds, "If you want twice the dose of omega-3s (600 mg) from the same sized pill as *Kirkland* [*Signature™*], you can spend 20 cents a pill for *Life Extension® Omega Foundations Super Omega-3 EPA/DHA With Sesame Lignans & Olive Extract*. If you want even more omega-3s without taking a second pill, we suggest *Solgar® Triple Strength Omega 3 950 mg* at 29 cents per softgel. These two products are our 'Top Picks' for high concentration fish oil."

As I was writing this book, ConsumerLab announced a new finding:

> If you want even more omega-3s without taking a second pill—and at even
> lower cost per 100 mg of EPA and DHA—we [now] suggest *Spring Valley*™
> [Walmart] *Maximum Care Omega-3 2000 mg*. Each softgel costs only 12
> cents and provides a whopping 955 mg of EPA and DHA. These two prod-
> ucts [from *Life Extension* and *Spring Valley*] are our "Top Picks" for high
> concentration fish oil. (Note: We added the *Spring Valley*™ *Maximum Care*
> product to this Review in January 2020 after a ConsumerLab reader spot-
> ted it on the market as a great deal and suggested that we test it. It replaces
> *Solgar Triple Strength Omega 3 950 mg* as a "Top Pick" because it provides
> similar amounts of omega-3s but at less than half the cost).

If you want an extremely concentrated fish oil to compete with the
prescription version, another of ConsumerLab's "Top Picks" is *Minami
Garden of Life® Platinum Omega-3 Fish Oil*. ConsumerLab writes, "Each
softgel provides 984 mg of EPA and DHA. However, each capsule is 70
cents [currently 75 cents]—much more expensive than others. This product provides a similar concentration and amount of omega-3s per capsule
as more expensive prescription fish oils such as Lovaza® . . . (and) it may
actually be better absorbed than Lovaza®."

However, an even better priced option is "*Viva® Naturals*, which provided 940 mg of EPA and DHA per softgel for only 17 cents [currently
19 cents]—less than one-third the cost of *Minami*." The current *Viva®
Naturals* fish oil is an "Ultra Strength Omega-3 Fish Oil" with 1880 mg
of EPA and DHA (1400 mg of EPA and 480 mg of DHA), which I found
online for as little as 22 cents per softgel.

The ConsumerLab review also includes information on omega-3 fatty
acids from other sources, such as algal oil, calamari oil, green-lipped mussel
oil, and krill oil. ConsumerLab does warn, "Note, however, that prescription drugs are held to higher standards than fish oil dietary supplements,
including the clinical demonstration of safety and efficacy and more rigorous manufacturing standards and oversight. This should be considered
when comparing products."

Other Natural Medicines for Hyperlipidemia

Red yeast rice is manufactured from rice on which a particular yeast has grown and produces cholesterol-lowering compounds that are a reddish color. It is a popular supplement in America, and *Natural Medicines* considers it "Possibly Effective" and "Likely Effective" for hyperlipidemia. They point out, "Clinical research shows that taking certain red yeast rice products (*Cholestin*®, Pharmanex; *Xuezhikang*®, Beijing Peking University; and others) 1–5 grams daily can significantly lower total cholesterol by 11 to 23 percent and low-density lipoprotein (LDL) cholesterol by 22 to 34 percent."

Also, "Most studies show that red yeast rice products can significantly decrease triglycerides and increase high-density lipoprotein (HDL) cholesterol in patients with hyperlipidemia. It may take up to 12 weeks to see the effects of red yeast rice on lipid parameters." But here's the catch: "These products provide up to 10–20 mg daily of monacolin K, which is identical to the 'statin' drug, lovastatin."

ConsumerLab warns, "In the late 1990s . . . the FDA determined that Cholestin®, by containing lovastatin, was an unapproved drug and ordered it removed from sale. A reformulated version of Cholestin®, containing no red yeast rice, is currently sold in the US. However, other red yeast rice dietary supplements continue to be sold in the US."

What about the other red yeast rice supplements? ConsumerLab advises, "The amount of lovastatins in the tested supplements ranged 1,500 percent. . . . When used according to their suggested serving sizes, only two of nine products provided amounts known to lower cholesterol in clinical trials. One of these two was half the price of the other, making it our 'Top Pick.'" ConsumerLab also found that lovastatin levels had fallen by 37 to 81 percent since 2014 in products it previously tested. This could result in decreasing efficacy."

Therefore, ConsumerLab warns, "Based on the varying amounts of lovastatins in products and decreases in these amounts over time, it may be preferable to use a prescription statin drug to ensure a more consistent dose (prescription lovastatin is also available at a lower cost than lovastatin from red yeast rice). However, red yeast rice may be effective for some people who don't respond to statin drugs and certain side effects may be diminished." A large study in Taiwan found that people who used red yeast rice (typical dose 600 mg containing 5.7 mg of monacolin K, taken twice daily) had a 54 percent lower risk of developing diabetes compared to people who used prescription lovastatin over five years.[39]

If you decide to take red yeast rice instead of a prescription statin, ConsumerLab's "Top Pick" is *HPF Cholestene*™. A serving of two capsules twice daily provides 12.9 mg of lovastatins—a dose likely to help lower elevated cholesterol levels. ConsumerLab says, "Comparing the cost to obtain 10 mg of lovastatins from each product, *HPF Cholestene*™ appears to provide the best value—just 49 cents per 10 mg, which is less than half the cost of getting the same amount of lovastatins from the next least expensive product, *Nature's Sunshine*®, at $1.03. The highest cost to get 10 mg of lovastatins is $7.60 from *Nature's Way*®."

However, in my area I can purchase prescription atorvastatin for as little as 7 cents for 10 mg and lovastatin for as little as 10 cents for 10 mg. This is 80 percent less than the lowest priced "Approved" or "USP®-Verified" red yeast rice products. And I'm guaranteed purity and consistency of product.

Natural Medicines concludes, "Don't recommend red yeast rice products due to product consistency issues and related safety concerns." I agree with that recommendation.

As for other popular natural medicines for hyperlipidemia, *Natural Medicines* tells doctors, "Due to questions about the effectiveness of garlic and policosanol, don't recommend them." Another wise caution is to "always remind patients about the importance of using treatments proven to reduce adverse cardiovascular outcomes (e.g., statins or pure EPA). Just because a drug or supplement reduces LDL cholesterol levels, this does not always equate to improved cardiovascular morbidity or mortality."

The following chart indicates the amazing number of natural medicines that have been evaluated for dyslipidemia. As you can see, the vast majority would either not be recommended or are not worth your money. But there are some safe and effective winners to consider. More detailed information is available from ConsumerLab.com and *Natural Medicines*.

Natural Medicines for Dyslipidemia, including Hypercholesterolemia and Hypertriglyceridemia

Safe / Effective	Likely Safe	Possibly Safe
Effective	★★★★★ • EPA (high TG) • EPA (Rx Vascepa/high TG) • Fish oil (high TG) • Fish oil (Rx Lovaza/high TG)	★★★
Likely Effective	★★★★ • Barley • Beta-glucans • Blond psyllium • Niacin • Oat bran • Plant stanols (Benecol Smart Chews or Softgels for high cholesterol) • Plant sterols (high cholesterol) • Sitostanol (high cholesterol)	★★ • Red yeast rice
Possibly Effective	★★★ • Avocado (high cholesterol) • Beta-sitosterol (high cholesterol) • Black currant • Broccoli (high cholesterol) • Calcium (high cholesterol) • Canola oil (high cholesterol) • Carob (high cholesterol) • Coffee • DASH diet • DHA (docosahexaenoic acid) • English walnuts (high cholesterol) • Flaxseed (high cholesterol) • Garlic • Green tea • Guar gum (high cholesterol) • Inulin (high TG) • Lactobacillus (high cholesterol) • Magnesium • N-acetyl cysteine (NAC)	★ • Artichoke • Berberine • Chromium • Gamma oryzanol • Glucomannan (high cholesterol) • Jiaogulan (high cholesterol) • Macadamia nut • Mesoglycan (high TG) • Pectin • Safflower (high cholesterol) • Sweet orange (high cholesterol)

| **Possibly Effective** | • Olive
• Probiotics (high cholesterol)
• Rice bran (high cholesterol)
• Selenium
• Soy
• Soybean oil (high cholesterol)
• Turmeric
• Vitamin C (high cholesterol)
• Yogurt | |

Insufficient evidence for safety or effectiveness AND/OR evidence for lack of safety or effectiveness

- Acacia (high cholesterol)
- Activated charcoal (high cholesterol)
- Alfalfa (high cholesterol)
- Algal oil
- Alpha-linolenic acid
- Amaranth (high cholesterol)
- Andrographis (high TG)
- Ashwagandha (high cholesterol)
- Astaxanthin (high cholesterol)
- Banana (high cholesterol)
- Beet (high TG)
- Bergamot
- Bifidobacteria
- Black currant seed oil
- Black seed
- Black tea
- Blue-green algae
- Borage seed oil
- Brewer's yeast (high cholesterol)
- Cabbage
- Casein protein
- Chitosan (high cholesterol)
- Chlorella
- Chokeberry (high cholesterol)
- Cocoa (high cholesterol)
- Coconut (high cholesterol)
- Cod liver oil (high cholesterol)
- Coenzyme Q10
- Colocynth
- Conjugated linoleic acid (CLA)
- Danshen
- Diatomaceous earth
- Dill
- Elderberry
- Evening primrose oil
- Fenugreek
- Fermented milk (high cholesterol)
- Fish oil
- Flaxseed oil
- Gamma-linolenic acid
- Ginger
- Glucosamine hydrochloride
- Grape
- Grapefruit (high cholesterol, high TG)
- Guggul
- Guggulipid
- Hazelnut
- Hesperidin (high cholesterol)
- Hibiscus
- Honey
- Hydroxymethylbutyrate (HMB)
- Hyperimmune egg
- Indian gooseberry (high cholesterol)
- Inositol nicotinate
- Inulin
- Irvingia gabonensis
- Job's tears
- Kefir (high cholesterol)
- Krill oil (dyslipidemia, high TG)
- Larch arabinogalactan
- L-arginine (high cholesterol)
- L-carnitine (dyslipidemia, high TG)
- Lecithin
- Lemongrass (high cholesterol)
- Licorice (high cholesterol)

- Lupin (high cholesterol)
- Lycopene
- Lysine (high TG)
- Macrobiotic diet
- Maritime pine (high cholesterol)
- Mediterranean diet
- Milk thistle (high cholesterol)
- Moringa
- Nattokinase
- Nicotinamide
- Nicotinamide riboside
- Organic food (high cholesterol)
- Paleo diet
- Pea protein
- Phaseolus vulgaris (high cholesterol)
- Plum (high cholesterol)
- Policosanol (high cholesterol)
- Pomegranate juice
- Prickly pear cactus (high cholesterol)
- Pyruvate
- Quercetin (high cholesterol)
- Quillaia (high cholesterol)
- Red clover
- Reishi mushroom
- Rhubarb (high cholesterol)
- Royal jelly
- Saccharomyces boulardii (high cholesterol)
- Sea buckhorn
- Sesame
- Sulfur
- Sweet almond (high cholesterol)
- Terminalia
- Theaflavin
- Tocotrienols (high cholesterol)
- Tree turmeric (high cholesterol)
- Vegetarian diet (high cholesterol)
- Vitamin B12 (high TG)
- Vitamin D
- Vitamin K (high cholesterol)
- Wheatgrass (high cholesterol)
- Whey protein
- White mulberry
- Yerba maté
- Yucca (high cholesterol)
- Zedoary (high cholesterol)

Most of the recommendations in the chart are based on the "Safety and Effectiveness Ratings" contained in *Natural Medicines™* and explained in chapter 4 of this book. They assume the use of high-quality, uncontaminated products and the use of typical doses. Keep in mind that some products are never appropriate for some patients due to concomitant disease states, potential drug interactions, or other clinical factors. Details are available at *Natural Medicines™*.

9

Energy and Fatigue

Energy Drinks and Shots

By this point in the book, you've learned that adequate sleep, a healthy and well-balanced diet, and regular exercise are the optimal ways to maintain your health and energy. However, most people have times when they feel they can benefit from an energy boost. Many supplements are widely advertised to help increase energy and decrease fatigue. As a result, energy drinks and shots have become hugely popular. Among adults, those eighteen to thirty-eight, particularly males, are the biggest consumers of energy drinks.[1]

Despite recent FDA scrutiny regarding the safety of these beverages, 2019 energy drink sales were up over 13 percent compared to 2018—up to almost $12 billion in US sales, including nearly $1 billion in sales of energy shots.[2] The National Center for Complementary and Integrative Health (NCCIH) reports, "Next to multivitamins, energy drinks are the most popular dietary supplement consumed by American teens and young adults."[3]

The terms *energy drink* and *energy shot* refer to caffeine-containing beverages that often have added vitamins, minerals, amino acids, or herbal mixtures. Besides providing high levels of caffeine, these drinks frequently contain

- added sugars;
- vitamins, particularly B vitamins;

111

- legal stimulants, such as guarana, a plant that grows in the Amazon;
- taurine, an amino acid that's in meat and fish;
- L-carnitine, a substance in our bodies that helps turn fat into energy (but does *not* "burn off" fat); and
- other popular ingredients including kola nut, ginkgo, and yerba maté.

Energy drinks are sold in containers and sizes similar to ordinary soft drinks, usually eight or sixteen ounces. The top-ten most popular energy drinks, based on 2019 sales, included products from *Red Bull®*, *Monster®*, *Bang®*, and *NOS®*.[4] *Red Bull®* has dominated energy drink sales, but "*Monster®* has experienced huge growth in the last few years."[5]

Energy shots are sold in small containers holding two to two and a half ounces of concentrated liquid. One product, *5-hour ENERGY®*, "has the 'energy shot' market cornered with none of the others anywhere in the same universe."[6]

However, in most cases, neither energy drinks nor energy shots deliver much real energy (i.e., calories). Instead what they provide is stimulation, primarily due to their significant caffeine content, including caffeine-containing plant products such as guarana or kola nut.

What about Caffeine?

Multiple studies over many years suggest real health benefits to drinking coffee. According to Johns Hopkins Medicine, caffeinated coffee has been linked with reduced risks for heart failure, stroke, type 2 diabetes, Parkinson's disease, Alzheimer's disease, and some types of cancer, such as colon and prostate cancer.[7] Recent studies have also found that coffee drinkers are less likely to die from some of the leading causes of death in women: coronary heart disease, stroke, diabetes, and kidney disease.[8]

Several sizeable studies have shown that people who drink moderate amounts of coffee (four to five eight-ounce cups) are less likely to die during the study period (between 10 and 15 percent less than non-coffee drinkers).[9] Coffee intake is associated with a lower risk of premature death. Another report explained that the "sweet spot appeared to be a coffee intake of 4–5 cups per day." At this level, men and women had a 12 percent and 16 percent respectively reduced risk of early death. Drinking six or more cups per day provided no additional benefit.

The report added, "However, even just one cup per day was associated with a five to six percent lowered risk of early death—showing that even a little bit is enough to have an effect."[10] The theory is that "since coffee is the number one source of antioxidants in the human diet,"[11] its antioxidants "might counteract the fundamental inflammatory mechanism associated with human aging."[12]

But just how much caffeine is safe? A 2019 study out of South Australia suggested "an upper limit of . . . five cups of coffee per day." Professor Elina Hyppönen, one of the study's authors, said, "To maintain a healthy heart and a healthy blood pressure, people must limit their coffees to fewer than six cups a day—based on our data six was the tipping point where caffeine started to negatively affect cardiovascular risk."[13] The study showed that once you reach six cups of coffee per day, the risk of heart disease increases by 22 percent.[14] Most coffee research defines a "cup of coffee" as eight ounces with an average of about 100 mg of caffeine per cup (although it can vary from 50 to 400 mg).[15]

According to the FDA, 400 mg per day or about four or five cups of coffee is the amount of caffeine "not generally associated with dangerous, negative effects" for healthy adults. Anything over that amount could potentially cause serious problems in adults and certainly children and adolescents. Although the amount of caffeine in over-the-counter products is limited to a maximum of 200 mg per dose, there is no limit for energy drinks.[16]

The American Medical Association (AMA) recommends healthy adults limit their caffeine intake to 500 mg a day.[17] But with energy drinks and shots, it can be challenging to tell how much you're ingesting as the labels on many of these products may be inaccurate.

According to a 2019 review by ConsumerLab.com, "*5-hour ENERGY*® lists among its ingredients an 'energy blend' that includes caffeine. The label notes that the amount of caffeine is comparable to that in a cup of 'leading premium coffee.'" ConsumerLab reported the 1.93 fluid ounce bottle contained 221.2 milligrams of caffeine, saying, "This is about 23 percent more than what you would get from a 'short' cup (eight fluid ounces) of a premium coffee such as Starbucks®, which Starbucks® claims to contain 180 mg of caffeine," or about 22.5 mg of caffeine per ounce. Many energy drinks and shots contain far more caffeine than this.

For example, in 2019, Caffeine Informer searched their database of over eight hundred energy products and reported on five products with more than 30 mg of caffeine per ounce:[18]

- *Redline® Xtreme Energy Drink* (39.5 mg)
- *SPIKE® Shooter* (35.7 mg)
- *Cocaine™ Energy Drink* (33.3 mg)
- *Redline® Princess* (31.3 mg)
- *Redline® Energy Drink* (31.3 mg)

In 2020, Caffeine Informer reported on two-ounce energy shots with the most caffeine:[19]

- *10-Hour Energy Shot* (422 mg)
- *Cocaine™ Energy Shot* (280 mg)
- *Phoenix Energy Shot* (280 mg)
- *7-Eleven® Energy Shot* (260 mg)
- *Rhino Rush Energy Shot* (250 mg)

This means you could exceed your 400 to 500 mg of caffeine per day with two eight-ounce servings of any of these drinks or one to two servings of these shots. There were another fourteen products containing between 15 and 30 mg of caffeine per ounce.

What about Added Sugars?

Besides the caffeine and vitamins in energy drinks, "a single 16-oz container of an energy drink may contain 54 to 62 grams of added sugar (equal to about 15 teaspoons of added sugar)," the NCCIH warns. "This exceeds the maximum amount of added sugars recommended for an entire day," which is six teaspoons per day for women and nine for men.[20]

It appears manufacturers and consumers are becoming more aware of this fact as the sale of sugar-free energy drinks is rapidly increasing. However, preliminary but "alarming research" from Canada reports, "Caffeinated energy drinks cause a 25 percent spike in teenagers blood glucose and insulin levels even when they contain no sugar." The researchers are concerned that in children and teens, "the caffeine alone in the drinks could predispose people to diabetes and heart disease."[21]

ConsumerLab also reviewed "nutrition bars & cookies—for energy, fiber, protein" in 2019, reporting they "can be a good source of real energy (calories), especially if you are on the go and haven't had a chance to eat a real meal, and also provide vitamins and minerals. It's important to choose carefully as some are high in sugar or contain sugar substitutes that may upset your stomach. Some also contain caffeine."

What about Stimulants and Vitamins?

Sheri Zidenberg-Cherr, PhD, vice chairwoman of the Department of Nutrition at the University of California, told CNN, "*5-hour ENERGY*® contains 200 milligrams [of caffeine] per serving, and keep in mind that does not include amounts of other stimulants found in energy drinks that can enhance the effects of caffeine."[22]

NCCIH explains that "guarana, commonly included in energy drinks, contains caffeine. Therefore, the addition of guarana increases the drink's total caffeine content."[23] And *Natural Medicines*™ warns, "Keep in mind that only the amount of ADDED caffeine must be stated on product labels. The amount of caffeine from caffeine-containing natural ingredients such as coffee or green tea does not need to be provided. This can make it difficult to determine the total amount of caffeine in a given product."

Energy drinks often contain B vitamins, such as B1 (thiamine), B2 (riboflavin), B3 (niacin), B6 (pyridoxine), and B9 (folic acid)—often much more than you need or want. Why the B vitamins? "Probably to try to sell you on the fact that B vitamins help convert food to energy," says ConsumerLab. "However, since few people are deficient in B vitamins, these added vitamins are likely to provide no benefit and may put you at risk for exceeding upper tolerable intake levels (ULs) for these vitamins—levels above which there is increasing risk of toxicity."

ConsumerLab adds, "Although many B vitamin supplements such as shot-sized energy drinks are touted as energy boosters, the real boost would appear to come from the often-unspecified amounts of caffeine added to many of these products."

Other Dangers of Energy Drinks and Shots

Should you use energy products? Are they safe? Studies show some of these products may help you stay alert or even improve athletic performance. However, researchers now believe that most of the positive effects of energy drinks on cognitive performance are related to the caffeine. Of course, caffeine can be found in many products (coffee, tea, or caffeine-only supplements). These products are also considered generally safe in most adults at less than 400 to 500 mg per day.[24]

The same is not true of energy drinks or shots due to many potential risks. Studies in military personnel found that frequent use (two times or more per day) or ingestion of more significant amounts (twenty-four ounces or more per day) of energy drinks was associated with a doubling or tripling of aggressive behaviors. Also, mental health problems (including sleep problems, depression, anxiety, post-traumatic stress disorder, and alcohol misuse) were significantly more common as compared to those who ingested no or few energy drinks. Interestingly, energy drink use was also associated with fatigue—likely due to inadequate sleep.[25]

NCCIH adds, "A growing body of scientific evidence shows that energy drinks can have serious health effects, particularly in children, teenagers, and young adults. In several studies, energy drinks have been found to improve physical endurance, but there's less evidence of any effect on muscle strength or power. Energy drinks may enhance alertness and improve reaction time, but they may also reduce steadiness of the hands."[26]

The American College of Sports Medicine (ACSM) adds, "Despite high market demand, the current evidence for safety, efficacy, and performance benefits is unsystematic and often contradictory, given different protocols and types of products consumed; this makes it difficult to draw firm conclusions. Also, much of the available literature is industry-sponsored."[27]

ConsumerLab points out, "The sugars in *Red Bull®* as well as [similar products] will also provide some quick energy. It's questionable, though, what all the other ingredients in these products bring to the table. There seems to be no good reason to have to deal with possible skin flush and tingling from all the niacin [vitamin B3] in just over one bottle of *5-hour ENERGY®* or a full bottle of *Rockstar®*—or liver injury from higher intakes." ConsumerLab points out that it's rare, but cases of acute hepatitis or nerve damage have been reported in otherwise healthy adults who consumed between 160 mg and 300 mg of niacin daily from energy drinks.

Energy drinks are also associated with increased cardiovascular issues. A study published in 2019 in *JAMA* found that caffeinated energy drinks altered the heart's electrical activity and raised blood pressure. The effects were "generally considered mild," according to study author Sachin Shah, PharmD, at the University of the Pacific. However, he added, "People who take certain medications or have a specific type of heart condition could be at increased risk of a fatal arrhythmia, or irregular heartbeat."[28] ConsumerLab also warns of unusual but potentially irreversible cases of nerve damage and imbalance as well as cases of gastrointestinal disturbances from excessive pyridoxine (vitamin B6) in energy drinks or shots.

John Higgins, MD, a sports cardiologist at the University of Texas Health Science Center in Houston who has led multiple studies on energy drinks and their health impact, said, "For certain groups, [energy drinks] could be potentially dangerous, like for

- those under 18,
- women who are pregnant,
- people who have a caffeine sensitivity,
- people who don't consume caffeine on a regular basis, and
- people who are taking certain medications, like Adderall for attention deficit (disorder)."[29]

According to NCCIH, "Between 2007 and 2011, the number of energy drink–related visits to emergency departments doubled. In 2011, one in ten of these visits resulted in hospitalization."[30] In 2016 there were more than twenty thousand emergency room visits attributable to the ingestion of energy drinks.[31]

An online survey of over two thousand adolescents and young adults (ages twelve to twenty-four) in Canada found that of those who had ever consumed an energy drink, about 55 percent had at least one adverse reaction. For 3 percent, the adverse reaction was bad enough they had either sought or considered seeking medical help. The most commonly reported reactions were rapid heartbeat (about 25 percent), difficulty sleeping (24 percent), headache (18 percent), nausea/vomiting/diarrhea (5 percent), and chest pain (3 percent). Additionally, energy drink consumers were almost three times more likely to report an adverse reaction than coffee consumers.[32] After reviewing the medical and poison control literature from around the world, Caffeine Informer listed fifteen possible dangers of consuming energy drinks:

1. Sudden death, cardiac arrest, abnormal heart contraction or arrythmia, high blood pressure, and reduction in the diameter of arteries
2. Headaches and migraines
3. Increased anxiety
4. Insomnia
5. Increased risk of type 2 diabetes (due to high sugar content)
6. Interaction with drugs or medications
7. Addiction
8. Risky behavior
9. Jitters or nervousness
10. Allergic reactions
11. Vomiting and other gastrointestinal side effects
12. Niacin (vitamin B3) overdose
13. Stress hormone release
14. Mental health problems and aggression
15. Fatigue[33]

The American Beverage Association stands by the safety of energy drinks, pointing out that many of their ingredients are also found in everyday foods and "have been rigorously studied for safety."[34] But health experts like the World Health Organization disagree, saying that energy drinks "may pose danger to public health."[35]

Who Should Avoid Energy Drinks?

The ACSM recommends, "Energy drinks should not be consumed by

- children or adolescents,
- pregnant or breastfeeding women,
- caffeine naïve or sensitive individuals,
- individuals taking stimulant or other caffeine-based medications, or
- those with certain cardiovascular or medical conditions."[36]

The National Federation of State High School Associations recommends that energy drinks not be used for hydration before, during, or after physical activity, adding, "Energy drinks are not sports drinks and should not be used by athletes in training or competition." They also caution, "Athletes taking over-the-counter or prescription medications should not consume energy drinks without the approval of their physician."[37]

Also, it is critically important not to mix energy drinks with alcohol. Caffeine can mask the depressant effects of alcohol and lead to dangerous situations in which a person may feel or act alert but be mentally compromised. The CDC warns that drinkers who consume alcohol mixed with energy drinks are more likely to binge drink, be taken advantage of or take advantage of someone else sexually, ride with a driver under the influence of alcohol, and sustain alcohol-related deaths or injuries.[38]

The NCCIH reports that about 25 percent of college students consume alcohol with energy drinks, and they binge drink significantly more often than students who don't mix them. Young drinkers who mix alcohol with energy drinks are four times more likely to binge drink at a high intensity (i.e., consume six or more drinks per binge episode) than drinkers who do not mix alcohol with energy drinks. The NCCIH reports that 42 percent of all energy drink–related emergency department visits involved combining these beverages with alcohol or drugs (such as marijuana or over-the-counter or prescription medicines).[39]

Caffeine Supplements

For caffeine supplements (not energy drinks or shots), *Natural Medicines* lists about 150 US and nearly 60 Canadian licensed products that are NMBER® rated 8 to 9 out of 10. Dr. Worthington points out, "Most of these products contain ~100–200 mg of caffeine, which is below the 400 mg daily level that is considered to be safe and is why they get the high NMBER value. However, consumers considering these products should keep in mind that these supplements might not be safe if the user is also consuming a significant amount of caffeine as part of their diet. Also, the NMBER rating applies to generally healthy adults and should not be applied to children/adolescents."

NSF® has "Certified" 66 caffeine-containing products from fifteen producers. ConsumerLab, USP®, and Labdoor have not evaluated any caffeine products.

Energy Bars

Although "Likely Safe," there's no evidence I'm aware of that "energy" bars actually increase energy. I can't recommend them for this indication. If you want to enjoy the convenience of an occasional bar for nutrition, ConsumerLab has these "Top Picks":

- fiber bar: *Fiber One Chewy Bars*—Oats & Chocolate
- high protein bar: *Pure Protein Bar*—Chewy Chocolate Chip
- meal replacement and food bar: *Probar Meal Superfood Slam*
- fruit and nut bar: *Larabar*—Cherry Pie, or *Kind*—Dark Chocolate Nuts & Sea Salt

But ConsumerLab warns, "Be aware that most of the bars provide at least 10 percent of the Daily Value of one or more vitamins or minerals. If you take vitamins or fortified products (such as fortified breakfast cereal) be careful not to exceed tolerable levels of vitamins and minerals." They add, "Also note that more than half of the fats in some bars (particularly those with high amounts of protein) are saturated ('bad') fats."

As for other natural medicines for energy, one of the most popular is *Panax ginseng. Natural Medicines* rates it as "Possibly Effective" for cognitive function for middle-aged people (but *not* young adults), but also, "'Possibly Unsafe' . . . when used orally, long-term . . . due to potential hormone-like effects which might cause adverse effects when used six months or more." I cannot recommend it for long-term use.

The Bottom Line

Caffeine, with the caveats mentioned above, is "Likely Safe" and "Likely Effective" for most adults. Unfortunately, the safety and effectiveness of energy drinks, shots, mixes, bars, and natural medicines are lacking. NCCIH reminds us, "A growing body of scientific evidence shows that energy drinks can have serious health effects, particularly in children, teenagers, and young adults."[40] This is complicated by the fact that the amount of caffeine in energy drinks varies widely and can be challenging to determine in some energy drinks. Whether they are sold as beverages or dietary supplements, there's no requirement that the amount of caffeine be listed on the label.

Many groups have advocated for regulatory limits on the caffeine content of energy drinks, as well as requiring labels to identify the actual amount of caffeine contained per serving.[41] Health Canada has already mandated changes to improve transparency and provide labels instructing vulnerable individuals to avoid energy drink use,[42] and it's time for the US to follow.

Mayo Clinic recommends, "For most people, occasional energy drinks are fine, but the amount of caffeine can vary from product to product. Try to limit yourself to no more than 400 milligrams of caffeine a day from all sources."[43] The experts at ConsumerLab agree, writing, "If you do choose to use any of these 'energy' products, it seems best to limit your daily intake and not consume any with high amounts of caffeine all at once. If you use these, avoid other caffeinated products or stimulants."

Mayo Clinic adds, "If you're consistently fatigued or run-down, however, consider healthier ways to boost your energy. Get adequate sleep, include physical activity in your daily routine, and eat a healthy diet. If these strategies don't seem to help, consult your doctor. Sometimes fatigue is a sign of an underlying medical condition, such as hypothyroidism or anemia. If you have an underlying condition such as heart disease or high blood pressure, ask your doctor if energy drinks may cause complications."[44]

Although I do not have the space to discuss the many other natural medicines that are peddled to increase energy and decrease fatigue, I've included ratings of the more common ones in the following chart. More detailed information can be obtained from ConsumerLab.com and *Natural Medicines*.

Natural Interventions and Medications to Increase Energy (Mental Alertness) and Decrease Fatigue

Safe / Effective	Likely Safe	Possibly Safe
Effective	★★★★★ • Regular exercise • Restful sleep	★★★
Likely Effective	★★★★ • Black tea • Caffeine • Coffee • Maintain a normal BMI • Mental stimulation • Oolong tea • Reduce stress	★★
Possibly Effective	★★★ • Acetyl-L-carnitine	★ • Energy bars • Pu-erh tea
Insufficient evidence for safety or effectiveness AND/OR evidence for lack of safety or effectiveness		
☹ • Aromatherapy • Astaxanthin • Basil • Bergamot • Black currant • Black pepper • Blue-green algae • Chlorella • Energy drinks • Energy shots • Guarana (short-term) • Ginkgo • Green tea • Iron	• Jasmine • Kola nut • Lavender • L-carnitine • Mangosteen • Massage • Panax ginseng • Reflexology • Rhodiola • Rosemary • Taurine • Theacrine • Vitamin B12 • White sandalwood (short-term) • Yerba maté	

Most of the recommendations in the chart are based on the "Safety and Effectiveness Ratings" contained in *Natural Medicines*™ and explained in chapter 4 of this book. They assume the use of high-quality, uncontaminated products and the use of typical doses. Keep in mind that some products are never appropriate for some patients due to concomitant disease states, potential drug interactions, or other clinical factors. Details are available at *Natural Medicines*™.

10

Gastrointestinal Health—Part 1

Probiotics and Digestive Enzymes

According to the NIH, sixty to seventy million Americans are affected by digestive diseases.[1] A 2019 survey from CRN reported that the age group most likely to purchase supplements for digestive health is thirty-five to fifty-four years—with 21 percent doing so.[2] Another 2019 survey, this one of internet users purchasing natural medicines to manage gastrointestinal (GI) symptoms, found that half (50 percent) were between the ages of twenty-six and forty-five, and a majority (88 percent) were women. Most participants (85 percent) reported the use of herbal supplements, and 85 percent of these used them not for general symptoms but a specific GI condition. The most common was gastroesophageal reflux (GERD, 44.4 percent).[3] These two surveys surprised me, as I would have guessed it was those fifty-five years of age and older using natural medicines for GI complaints.

Some of the more common GI difficulties for which people use natural medicines include (in alphabetical order)

- bloating and gas,
- celiac disease (which includes gluten sensitivity and gluten intolerance),

- chronic recurrent abdominal pain (CRAP),
- constipation,
- diarrhea,
- diverticulosis and diverticulitis,
- gallstones,
- GERD,
- hemorrhoids,
- inflammatory bowel disease (IBD, including Crohn's disease [CD] and ulcerative colitis [UC]), and
- irritable bowel syndrome (IBS).

An entire book would be needed to address all of these, so let me first emphasize some of the natural medicines used for the more common GI difficulties. Then we'll switch gears and quickly review the evidence for and against considering natural medicines for several specific digestive difficulties.

Probiotics

One article says the food we eat exposes "our insides to billions of different bacteria in addition to those we were born with. Many of those minuscule creatures play important roles—good and bad—in how well we absorb nutrients, the functionality of our immune response, and our energy and metabolism levels." Furthermore, "As we age, the types and amount of microbes found in the gut are reduced. As the diversity of bacteria diminishes, a process called *inflamm-aging* occurs, contributing to age-related inflammatory processes that can lead to cancer, neurological disorders, and other diseases."[4]

According to *Harvard Health*, "An estimated 100 trillion microorganisms representing more than 500 different species inhabit every normal, healthy bowel. These microorganisms (or microflora) generally don't make us sick; most are helpful. Gut-dwelling bacteria keep pathogens (harmful microorganisms) in check, aid digestion and nutrient absorption, and contribute to immune function."[5]

The Academy of Nutrition and Dietetics (AND) says, "Prebiotics are naturally occurring, nondigestible food components that are linked to promoting the growth of helpful bacteria in your gut. Simply said, they're 'good' bacteria promoters. Prebiotics include fructooligosaccharides, such as inulin and galactooligosaccharides. But rather than focusing on these lengthy words, include more prebiotics in your day by eating more fruits, vegetables, and whole grains such as bananas, onions, garlic, leeks, asparagus, artichokes, beans, and whole-grain foods."[6]

Probiotics (from *pro* and *biota*, meaning "for life") contain live microorganisms (bacteria and yeasts). AND advises, "To include more probiotics in your eating plan, look to fermented dairy foods including yogurt, kefir products, and aged cheeses, which contain live cultures [of 'good bacteria'] such as bifidobacteria and lactobacillus. Also consider fermented, non-dairy foods with beneficial live cultures, including kimchi, sauerkraut, miso, tempeh, and cultured non-dairy yogurts."[7]

AND adds, "Ultimately, prebiotics, or 'good' bacteria promoters, and probiotics, the 'good' bacteria, work together synergistically. In other words, prebiotics are breakfast, lunch, and dinner for probiotics, which restores and can improve GI health. Products that combine these together are called *synbiotics*."[8]

"In addition to foods traditionally prepared with live bacterial cultures . . . consumers can now purchase probiotic capsules and pills, fruit juices, cereals, sausages, cookies, candy, [and] granola bars," writes *Scientific American*. "Indeed, the popularity of probiotics has grown so much in recent years that manufacturers have even added the microorganisms to cosmetics and mattresses."[9]

In its 2020 Survey of Supplement Users, ConsumerLab.com reported probiotics were the sixth most popular natural medicine in the US, taken by about 39 percent of those who take supplements. According to the most recent NIH survey, the number of adults in the US taking probiotics or their cousins, prebiotics (typically nondigestible fibers that favor the development of gut bacteria), has more than quadrupled to nearly four million.[10] AGA writes, "The probiotics industry is growing rapidly, with sales in the United States alone expected to exceed $6 billion in 2020."[11] One research firm estimates that the global probiotics market exceeded 35 billion USD in 2015 and predicts that it will reach 66 billion by 2024.[12]

Why are probiotics so popular? One group of researchers may provide a clue: "In the current era where distrust in medical experts and health authorities is widespread, individual consumption of over-the-counter health products is largely guided by information collected on the Internet."[13] But as I mentioned earlier, the internet is not a particularly good place to look for trustworthy, evidence-based information. Apparently, this is especially true when it comes to probiotics. *Scientific American* advises, "A closer look at the science underlying microbe-based treatments, however, shows that most of the health claims for probiotics are pure hype."[14]

For example, a 2020 study from European researchers reported, "Most websites that provide information about probiotics are unreliable and often tout unproven health benefits." The investigators found that most probiotic websites were commercial ones, "hoping to sell a product," while "others were news sites or health portals (providing links to other sites)." They concluded, "Commercial websites on average provide the least reliable information, and significant numbers of claimed benefits of probiotics are not supported by scientific evidence." Furthermore, only one in four of the websites mentioned any potential side effects from taking probiotics.[15]

AGA concluded, "Probiotics are a source of significant cost with unclear benefit."[16] An expert in the study of the healthy human gut microbiota, both in disease and in health, Professor Emma Allen-Vercoe, PhD, at the University of Guelph in Canada says, "For the most part, the claims that are made are enormously inflated."[17] *Scientific American* writes, "The majority of studies to date have failed to reveal any benefits in individuals who are already healthy. The bacteria seem to help only those people suffering from a few specific intestinal disorders."[18] Matthew A. Ciorba, MD, a gastroenterologist at Washington University in St. Louis, agrees, saying, "There is no evidence to suggest that people with normal gastrointestinal tracts can benefit from taking probiotics. If you're not in any distress, I would not recommend them."[19] But, with all that said, certain specific probiotics may be helpful to some people with particular conditions.

If you are going to try them for a particular disorder, it's critical to understand that not all probiotics are the same. Different strains of bacteria or yeast can have completely different effects. In other words, if you just go to the store and buy any probiotic, there's no guarantee that the types of bacteria listed on a label are useful for the condition you want to take them for. Any of the health benefits of probiotics are strain specific.

Dr. Worthington explains, "When we say, 'strain-specific,' it doesn't just mean the same species. Even among the same species of probiotics, there are differences among strains. For instance, *Lactobacillus rhamnosus* GR-1, in combination with *Lactobacillus reuteri* RC-1461, has shown some benefit for UTI and vaginosis. On the other hand, *Lactobacillus rhamnosus GG* (which is different from GR-1) has value in treating diarrhea (various causes), atopic disease, and URTI. And *Lactobacillus reuteri* DSM 17938 (which differs from RC-1461) has shown benefit for constipation and diarrhea."

Dr. Worthington adds, "Not only do different species/strains seem to have different effects, there is some evidence that combinations of probiotics work differently than single strains. In some disorders, the combinations seem to work better than single species/strains. But for other conditions (e.g., antibiotic-associated diarrhea), the combinations seem to work only as well or possibly less well than single strains."

But when it comes to quality testing, ConsumerLab has some good news: "Among the [23] probiotic supplements for people selected by Consumer-Lab for testing, most passed testing, but a liquid probiotic [*Mary Ruth's® Liquid Probiotic—Unflavored*] was discovered to be contaminated with a pathogenic bacteria [and] capsules of another probiotic [*NewRhythm® Probiotics 50 Billion CFU*] failed to live up to their claim of being enteric-coated. All of the other 21 products selected for testing by ConsumerLab provided the amounts of probiotics listed on their labels and met the other requirements relating to quality. An additional 13 products passed the same testing in ConsumerLab's Quality Certification Program."

This is a distinct improvement from previous tests of probiotics by ConsumerLab that found a much larger percentage of products that "did not contain their claimed amounts of viable cells, suggesting that many manufacturers have improved their products and/or improved the conditions under which the products are shipped and stored prior to purchase."

However, many commercially available probiotics are not helpful for *any* indication, while others may be harmful. I recommend you consult a health professional familiar with probiotics or use the extensive resources at ConsumerLab or *Natural Medicines*™ to investigate your best options.

Digestive Enzymes

Digestive enzymes are produced primarily in the pancreas gland. For example, lipase breaks down fats, amylase dissolves carbohydrates, and proteases or peptidases cleave proteins. They all help digest food so we can absorb nutrients. Our mouth, stomach, and small intestine also produce some digestive enzymes. They are great for our health.

Pancreatic enzyme products that are available by prescription (*Creon*®, e.g.) are safe and effective in some people with specific types of pancreatic insufficiency. However, as Dr. Worthington warns, "Supplements containing the same enzymes as these prescription products are also available, but they are not the same. All prescription formulations are derived from porcine pancreas, contain standardized and consistent amounts of pancrelipase, and may be enteric-coated. Supplemental forms of pancreatic enzyme products also contain lipase, amylase, and protease enzymes; however, unlike the prescription products, the amount of active ingredient in pancreatic enzyme supplements can vary from one batch to the next." In other words, the prescription and supplement enzymes, although appearing the same, are as different as night and day.

According to the *Washington Post*, "Promotions for some of these supplements do more than promise they will cure digestive ailments. They also claim the supplements will help people lose weight, think more clearly, and even give people the ability to eat foods they're allergic to."[20] *Harvard Health* advises, "Digestive enzyme supplements promise to fix everything from bloating and flatulence to heartburn and gut health. The supplements are so popular that global sales are expected to reach $1.6 billion [USD] by 2025 . . . but don't be too quick to reach for them." Dr. Kyle Staller, MD, MPH, a gastroenterologist at Harvard-affiliated Massachusetts General Hospital, says, "Some of them are clearly beneficial, in certain situations.

But enzyme supplements also are often used in situations where there is little evidence that they do any good."[21]

Historically, the most popular digestive enzyme is *Beano®*. It's been around since the early 1990s, long before digestive enzymes started trending, and breaks down the carbohydrates in beans into simpler sugars to make them easier to digest—and less likely to produce gas. Another common digestive enzyme is lactase, which breaks down lactose, a natural sugar found in milk. If you don't produce enough lactase, the undigested lactose travels into the colon, causing cramping, gas, and diarrhea that are hallmarks of lactose intolerance. Lactase pills—or lactose-free milk products (e.g., *Lactaid®*), which have the enzyme already added—can prevent the symptoms. Of course, people with these problems can just avoid those foods, but in these specific situations, these particular supplements can be both safe and effective.

Nevertheless, for those choosing to try a digestive enzyme, ConsumerLab has tested twelve, of which eleven were "Approved." They write, "If you are looking for an all-around digestive enzyme supplement of high quality with substantial activity in digesting carbohydrates and fats, as well as some protein action, four products stand out based on our analyses:

- *Pure Encapsulations® Digestive Enzymes Ultra* (62 cents per 2-capsule serving),
- *Enzymedica® Digest Gold™ with ATPro* (40 cents per 1-capsule serving),
- *Doctor's Best® Digestive Enzymes* (22 cents per 1 veggie cap serving), and
- *Healthy Origins® Digestive Enzymes* (16 cents per 1 veggie cap serving)."

ConsumerLab's "Top Pick" is *Healthy Origins® Digestive Enzymes*. Now, let's dive into some of the more common GI conditions.

11

Gastrointestinal Health—Part 2

Celiac Disease, Irritable Bowel Syndrome, and Inflammatory Bowel Disease

Celiac Disease

Celiac disease, sometimes called *celiac sprue* or *gluten-sensitive enteropathy*, is an immune reaction to eating gluten, a protein found in wheat, barley, and rye. If you have celiac disease, eating gluten can trigger an immune response in your small intestine. Over time, this reaction damages your small intestine's lining and prevents it from absorbing some nutrients (malabsorption). The intestinal damage often causes diarrhea, fatigue, weight loss, bloating, and anemia and can lead to serious complications.

The Celiac Disease Foundation says, "It is estimated to affect 1 in 100 people worldwide. Two and one-half million Americans are undiagnosed and are at risk for long-term health complications." They add, "There's no cure for celiac disease—but for most people, following a strict gluten-free diet can help manage symptoms and promote intestinal healing."[1] The foundation has great resources at www.celiac.org.

Up to 30 percent of people with celiac will continue with symptoms even on a strict gluten-free diet. Many turn to natural medicines for this.

Prescriber's Letter™ advises, "Patients with celiac disease often try probiotics despite insufficient evidence of efficacy for disease symptoms." They tell prescribers to "caution patients that probiotics may contain gluten, even those with labeling to the contrary."[2] (Fortunately, ConsumerLab.com and LabDoor both test natural medicines for gluten. You can read more about gluten-free fiber in the section "High Fiber Foods for Dyslipidemia" in chapter 8.)

Natural Medicines™ was only able to identify studies looking at bifidobacteria, inulin, and L-carnitine in the treatment of celiac disease and rated all as "Insufficient Evidence" of effectiveness.[3] A 2020 meta-analysis of six studies published in the *American Journal of Gastroenterology* concluded, "Patients with celiac disease who adhere to a gluten-free diet and use probiotics may experience improvements in gastrointestinal symptoms; [however], the overall certainty of the evidence ranged from very low to low."[4]

At this point in time, there are no natural medicines I can recommend to my patients for celiac disease.

In regard to gluten-free diets, the *Harvard Health Letter* advises, "It's important to know that it can set you up for some nutritional deficiencies. . . . This can be a problem for anyone, but it's especially worrisome for children and women who are pregnant or may become pregnant."[5]

Physician and registered dietitian Amy Burkhart writes, "Awareness has increased regarding common vitamin and nutrient deficiencies on a gluten-free diet. Common deficiencies include vitamin D, iron, B vitamins, calcium, zinc, copper, and vitamins A, E, and K." She adds, "Gluten-free dieters are taking [supplements] to prevent possible deficiencies or address persistent symptoms. Supplements can be beneficial, but they need to be used with caution." If you're on a gluten-free diet, I recommend her article "Four Vitamin Toxicities on a Gluten-Free Diet" at tinyurl.com/y4 yesj33. *US News* has a nice review on the gluten-free diet at tinyurl.com /y4wkps5m.

Should you consider a gluten-free diet if you don't have celiac disease? The *Harvard Health letter* reports, "Based on little or no evidence other than testimonials in the media, people have been switching to gluten-free diets to lose weight, boost energy, treat autism, or generally feel healthier."[6]

Mayo Clinic advises, "A gluten-free diet is recommended for some specific medical reasons, including celiac disease and gluten sensitivity. Beyond this, there's little evidence that a gluten-free diet offers any particular health benefits, but it can be a healthy way to eat, depending on your food choices."[7]

The gluten-free diet for general health doesn't make much sense to Dr. Daniel A. Leffler, director of clinical research at the Celiac Center at Beth Israel Deaconess Medical Center in Boston. He says, "People who are sensitive to gluten may feel better, but a larger portion will derive no significant benefit from the practice. They'll simply waste their money, because these products are expensive."[8]

I do not recommend a gluten-free diet for people without celiac disease or sensitivity.

Irritable Bowel Syndrome (IBS)

IBS is a widespread GI disorder, affecting between 10 and 15 percent of Americans, that causes chronic recurrent abdominal discomfort and bloating associated with altered bowel habits. IBS with predominant diarrhea is called *IBS-D*, with mainly constipation is called *IBS-C*, and with alternating bouts of both is called *mixed IBS* or *IBS-M*. IBS is the most common disease diagnosed by gastroenterologists and one of the most common disorders seen by primary care physicians. It is also the second most common reason for work absence after the common cold.[9]

The American College of Gastroenterology (ACG) recommends exercise (weak evidence), fiber (moderate-to-strong evidence), and several pharmaceuticals for IBS (moderate-to-strong evidence), but the prescriptions can be costly.[10] According to ConsumerLab, "Non-pharmaceutical interventions for IBS—notably the low FODMAP diet, cognitive behavioral therapy, and gut-directed hypnotherapy—have performed well in clinical trials, but the time and commitment they require can be difficult for some people."

In fact, because of the increasing research into the potent "brain-gut connection," there's a new and growing field called *psychogastroenterology*, "in which trained psychologists and clinical social workers are employing a variety of interventions aimed at improving communications between the gut and brain. This is achieved in various ways: retrain the brain to properly interpret signals from the gut [and] help people who have long suffered from [IBS] to break some of their learned thought and behavior patterns that can feed the vicious cycle of a dysfunctional brain-gut interaction."[11]

However, because of the costs and side effects of these recommended therapies, many people try natural medicines instead of or in combination with traditional treatments. Here are some to consider.

BLOND PSYLLIUM. *Natural Medicines* reports that blond psyllium is "Likely Safe" and "Effective" in treating constipation and "Possibly Effective" in treating diarrhea and IBS. For IBS, most experts recommend slowly working up to 20 to 30 grams of fiber a day. For more information about blond psyllium or fiber, see the appendix.

SENNA. Another fiber product, senna (*Senekot®*, which is an FDA-approved nonprescription drug), is "Likely Safe" and "Likely Effective" for short-term use for constipation. However, it is "Possibly Unsafe" when taken long-term or in high doses. *Natural Medicines* advises, "Don't use senna for more than two weeks. Longer use can cause the bowels to stop functioning normally and might cause dependence on laxatives."

PEPPERMINT OIL. *Natural Medicines* reports, "Several clinical trials and meta-analyses show that taking enteric-coated peppermint oil 1–2 capsules orally three times daily reduces abdominal pain, distention, flatulence, and bowel movements in patients with IBS." The most recent meta-analysis to date shows that in patients with IBS, peppermint oil reduced abdominal pain in about one-half and persistent IBS symptoms in about one-third of them. They add, "Most trials have used specific peppermint oil products (*Colpermin*™, Tillotts Pharma [26 cents per capsule]; *Mintoil*, Cadigroup; *IBgard®*, IM Healthscience [57 cents per capsule])." *Natural Medicines* lists dozens of peppermint oil products NMBER® rated 9 out of 10, including *Colpermin*™, and several rated 8 out of 10, including *IBgard®*. Consumer-Lab, USP®, and Labdoor have not evaluated peppermint products.

BIFIDOBACTERIA. An option suggested by *Natural Medicines* is the probiotic bifidobacteria. They write,

> Various Bifidobacteria-containing probiotics have been evaluated for improving gastrointestinal symptoms in patients with IBS. The best evidence is for a specific Bifidobacterium strain called *Bifidobacterium infantis* 35624

(*Align*® [NMBER 8 out of 10, 96 cents per day]). Consuming this product in daily doses of 100 million colony-forming units as capsules or 1 billion colony-forming units as a malted milk drink for four to eight weeks reduces abdominal pain, bloating, and bowel movement difficulty in patients with IBS. Improvement is seen within one week of treatment.

Other clinical research shows that taking a specific bifidobacteria strain called *Bifidobacterium lactis B19* (10 billion colony-forming units daily for four weeks) also reduces bloating, feelings of abdominal fullness, and difficulty with defecation in 25 to 50 percent of patients with IBS.

OTHER PROBIOTICS. There is a wide variation in dosing depending on the strain of lactobacillus or bifidobacteria used. *Natural Medicines* reports, "A specific product containing heat-killed *Lactobacillus acidophilus* (*Lactéol*® *Fort*), a specific beverage containing *Lactobacillus plantarum* 299v (*ProViva*), or capsules containing *Lactobacillus plantarum* 299v have been used for 4 weeks. *Saccharomyces* [*boulardii* CNCM I-745] (*Bioflor*®) 200 billion colony-forming units daily for 4 weeks has been used."

Natural Medicines adds, "Some research has evaluated bifidobacteria in combination with other probiotic species. One clinical study shows that a specific combination probiotic containing strains of lactobacillus, bifidobacterium, and streptococcus (i.e., *VSL#3*®) decreases bloating in patients with diarrhea-predominant IBS."

ConsumerLab advises, "*Visbiome*® *High Potency Probiotic* (by ExeGi Pharma and also referred to as the 'original De Simone formulation' after its inventor) is the original *VSL#3* formula that was used in many clinical trials. Due to legal disputes, what is now sold as *VSL#3*® *The Living Shield* (by Pharmaceuticals/Alfasigma and distributed in the US by Sigma-Tau Healthscience USA) is not the original." In addition, "Be aware that there are concerns about taking the probiotic currently sold as *VSL#3* around the time of surgery."

The *Visbiome*® product is ConsumerLab's "Top Pick" for IBS. They advise, "*Visbiome*® *High Potency Probiotic* ($1.67 per 2 capsules providing a total of 225 billion cells) may reduce bloating in diarrhea-predominant IBS—although it may not improve other symptoms such as abdominal pain, gas, and urgency. About 4 capsules are taken twice daily."

Natural Medicines lists over two dozen products containing bifidobacteria that are NMBER rated 8 out of 10, including *Align®* and *Bifantis®*. *Natural Medicines* does not have a NMBER rating for *Visbiome®* or *VSL#3®*. Labdoor gave an "A-minus" rating to *Align®*.

Of interest, a 2020 Clinical Practice Guideline by the American Gastroenterological Association (AGA) concluded, "In symptomatic children and adults with irritable bowel syndrome, we recommend the use of probiotics only in the context of a clinical trial." They add, "The overall quality of evidence was very low. . . . Although there has been significant interest and potential for the use of probiotics in IBS, further studies are needed to clarify this important question."[12]

Nevertheless, as Dr. Worthington writes, "IBS is a condition for which many probiotics have been studied, but only certain types of probiotic formulations provide benefit for IBS symptoms."

As listed in the chart at the end of the chapter, many other natural medicines are promoted for IBS but cannot be recommended. But my application of all the information above leads me to recommend four probiotic products. I usually start with *Align®* for IBS and *Visbiome®* for IBS-D. If these don't help, I'll next try *Bioflor®* or *Bifantis®*.

Inflammatory Bowel Disease (IBD)

Inflammatory bowel disease (IBD) is a term that describes chronic inflammatory disorders of the GI tract that can cause severe diarrhea, abdominal pain, bloody stools, fever and fatigue, and weight loss. In the US, over three million individuals have IBD. Two forms are most common:

- ulcerative colitis (UC), which causes superficial ulcers in the large intestine (colon) and rectum
- Crohn's disease (CD), which causes deep ulcers anywhere from the mouth to the anus, although they are most common in the small intestine

IBD is a complex chronic condition with no cure that is very difficult to treat. Furthermore, conventional treatments can be costly and have significant side effects. As a result, "As many as half of all patients with IBD use some form of natural medicine," says *Natural Medicines*, "to find relief they haven't found with conventional medicines, to reduce the expense of conventional medicines, and to avoid the side effects of conventional medicines."

Natural Medicines adds, "Many . . . use natural medicines in addition to conventional therapy. Others don't like using conventional medications for IBD, especially steroids. These patients are particularly concerning because they often end up using natural medicines instead of conventional medications." *Natural Medicines* writes to health professionals,

> Several natural medicines show promise in treating ulcerative colitis: andrographis, blond psyllium, Indian frankincense [boswellia], and some probiotic species. Many clinical studies support their use, but many details on optimum dose, duration, and how to combine them with conventional treatments are still needed. Other natural medicines show preliminary evidence for treating ulcerative colitis or Crohn's disease . . . including fish oil and turmeric, [which] are popular. However, until more is known, it's too early to recommend these for IBD.
>
> Lastly, it's important to remember that not all natural medicines are harmless. Help patients steer clear of natural medicines which may aggravate IBD or interact with conventional medications used to treat IBD. [For instance, concomitant use of turmeric can increase levels of the prescription drug sulfasalazine, which is often used to treat UC.]

The 2020 AGA Clinical Practice Guideline concludes that in adults and children with ulcerative colitis or Crohn's disease, the use of probiotics should occur only in the context of a clinical trial. Even though there have been a number of published studies, "the overall quality of the evidence was rated as low." AGA adds, "Further studies are needed to define specific populations of patients with Crohn's disease who might benefit from probiotics, as well as the most effective probiotic strains."[13]

The Bottom Line

If you have IBD, follow all the recommendations of your gastroenterologist. If you want to add natural medicines to your conventional therapy, be sure to both carefully research your options on ConsumerLab or *Natural*

Medicines and discuss the options with your gastroenterologist before starting.

Because of space constraints, I can't discuss all of the options you might consider. Nevertheless, I've summarized in the following charts those that are commonly used. Complete details on any of these substances can be found at ConsumerLab.com and *Natural Medicines*.

Natural Interventions and Medications for Celiac Disease

Safety / Effective	Likely Safe	Possibly Safe
Likely Effective	★★★★★ • Gluten-free diet	★★★
Possibly Effective	★★★	★
Insufficient evidence for safety or effectiveness AND/OR evidence for lack of safety or effectiveness		
☹ • Bifidobacteria • Inulin • L-carnitine • Probiotics		

Natural Medicines for Irritable Bowel Syndrome (IBS)

Safety / Effective	Likely Safe	Possibly Safe
Effective	★★★★★ • Blond psyllium (constipation)	★★★
Likely Effective	★★★★ • Peppermint oil (enteric-coated) • Probiotics (especially bifidobacteria) • Align • Bifantis • Duolac Care • Visbiome • Senna (short term, constipation)	★★ • Cascara (IBS-C) • European buckthorn (IBS-C)

Safety / Effective	Likely Safe	Possibly Safe
Possibly Effective	★★★ • Blond psyllium (diarrhea) • Karaya gum • Probiotics • Lactéol fort • Wheat bran	★ • Aloe (IBS-C) • Fermented milk
Insufficient evidence for safety or effectiveness AND/OR evidence for lack of safety or effectiveness		
☹ • Agrimony (IBS-D) • Artichoke • Blackberry leaf (IBS-D) • Black tea (IBS-D) • Clown's mustard plant • Cultura • Culturelle • Fenugreek • Fish oil • Flaxseed • Ginger • Horse chestnut	• Melatonin • Oak bark (IBS-D) • Pectin • Probiotics • ProViva • Quebracho • Raspberry leaf (IBS-D) • Reflexology • Rhubarb (IBS-C) • Turmeric • VSL#3 • Yoga	

Natural Medicines for Inflammatory Bowel Disease (IBD), including Crohn's Disease (CD) and Ulcerative Colitis (UC)

Safety / Effective	Likely Safe	Possibly Safe
Effective	★★★★★	★★★
Likely Effective	★★★★	★★★
Possibly Effective	★★★ • Andrographis (UC) • Blond psyllium (UC) • Boswellia (Indian frankincense for UC) • Probiotics • VSL#3 (UC)	★★★ • Phosphatidylcholine (UC)

Insufficient evidence for safety or effectiveness AND/OR evidence for lack of safety or effectiveness

☹

- Aloe gel (UC)
- Alpha-linolenic acid
- Barley (UC)
- Beta-glucans
- Blond psyllium (CD)
- Boswellia (Indian frankincense for CD)
- Bromelain (UC)
- Conjugated linoleic acid
- Culturelle (CD)
- DHA
- EPA
- Evening primrose oil (UC)
- Fish oil (CD, UC)
- Gamma-linolenic acid (UC)
- Glutamine (CD)
- Green tea (UC)
- Iron
- Lactobacillus (CD)
- N-acetyl glucosamine
- Oats
- Peppermint
- Probiotics
- Rutin
- Turmeric (CD, UC)
- Vitamin A
- Vitamin B6 (pyridoxine)
- Vitamin B12 (cobalamin)
- Vitamin E
- Wheat bran
- Wheatgrass (UC)
- Zinc

The recommendations in the charts are based almost entirely on the "Safety and Effectiveness Ratings" contained in *Natural Medicines*™ and explained in chapter 4 of this book. They assume the use of high-quality, uncontaminated products and the use of typical doses. Keep in mind that some products are never appropriate for some patients due to concomitant disease states, potential drug interactions, or other clinical factors. Details are available at *Natural Medicines*™.

12

Gastrointestinal Health—Part 3

Diarrhea, Constipation, and Indigestion

Most people have no idea how large their digestive system really is. For example, about sixty tons of food pass through it during the average lifetime.[1] The small intestine, which does most of the work of digestion using enzymes and absorbing nutrients for the body to use, is about twenty-two feet long and about one inch in diameter. Based upon that, you'd expect the surface area of the small intestine to be about six square feet—but due to its fantastic design features, including two to ten billion tiny villi—its surface area is actually around 2,700 square feet or about the size of a tennis court.

Your gastrointestinal (GI) tract is closely connected to your brain by nerves, hormones, and even the immune system.[2] Emotions (including stress) and brain disorders can dramatically affect your digestive system. Your liver, spleen, and pancreas are your second-, seventh-, and eighth-largest organs, respectively. And did you know your body can move your food through the digestive system even while you are hanging upside down? It does not depend upon gravity because it works with muscles. In this chapter we'll cover some of the most common GI complaints and popular natural medicines used to treat them.

Acute Infectious Diarrhea (Gastroenteritis or Stomach Flu)

Researchers estimate that about 179 million cases of acute diarrhea occur in the US each year.[3] *Natural Medicines*™ writes, "There is some clinical evidence that probiotics have a role in preventing and treating diarrhea from all causes. The best evidence is for *Saccharomyces boulardii*. Research also shows that lactobacillus-containing probiotic preparations can prevent and treat diarrhea in certain patients. Clinical research on the use of probiotic-containing yogurt for diarrhea treatment and prevention is mixed."

The 2017 Infectious Diseases Society of America (IDSA) guidelines recommend probiotics as an option for reducing symptoms of diarrhea. They point out that two specific strains, *Lactobacillus GG* (*Culturelle*® is the best studied) and *Saccharomyces boulardii* (*Florastor*® is used in most studies) have been shown to shorten the course of infectious diarrhea.[4]

The AGA guidelines say, "The majority of the data supporting the use of probiotics in children with acute infectious gastroenteritis were from studies performed outside of the US and Canada, while two high-quality studies performed in the US and Canada did not show any benefit." For acute infectious gastroenteritis, the AGA suggests "against the use of probiotics."[5]

In my practice, I do not recommend probiotics for acute gastroenteritis (stomach flu).

Travelers' Diarrhea

Gastroenterologist and travel medicine expert Bradley A. Connor, MD, writes, "Travelers' diarrhea (TD) is the most predictable travel-related illness. Attack rates range from 30 to 70 percent of travelers, depending on the destination and season of travel. Traditionally, it was thought that TD could be prevented by following simple recommendations such as 'boil it, cook it, peel it, or forget it,' but studies have found that people who follow these rules may still become ill. Poor hygiene practice in local restaurants is likely the largest contributor to the risk for TD."[6]

There is increasing interest in natural medicines to prevent travelers' diarrhea as, in 2019, the CDC advised, "At this time, prophylactic antibiotics should not be recommended for most travelers. Prophylactic antibiotics afford no protection against nonbacterial pathogens and can remove normally protective microflora from the bowel. This increases the risk of infection with resistant bacterial pathogens. . . . Additionally, prophylactic antibiotics limit the therapeutic options if TD occurs." Instead, they advise "prompt, early self-treatment with antibiotics when moderate to severe TD occurs,"[7] which means taking the antibiotic with you on your trip but not starting it until you have TD and it's worsening.

Dr. Connor writes, "The primary [non-prescription] agent studied for prevention of TD, other than antimicrobial drugs, is bismuth subsalicylate (BSS), which is the active ingredient in adult formulations of *Pepto-Bismol*® and *Kaopectate*®. Studies from Mexico have shown that this agent (taken daily as either 2 ounces of liquid or 2 chewable tablets 4 times per day) reduces the incidence of TD by approximately 50 percent. . . . Travelers with aspirin allergy and those taking anticoagulants should not take BSS. In travelers taking aspirin or salicylates for other reasons, the use of BSS may result in salicylate toxicity."[8]

Clinical guidelines published by ACG in 2016 give a strong recommendation for the use of BSS to control and prevent mild to moderate travelers' diarrhea. *Natural Medicines* advises, "The salicylate part of [BSS] has anti-diarrheal effects. . . . The bismuth moiety has anti-bacterial and anti-viral properties and is involved in the prevention of diarrhea." They add, "When used prophylactically, [it] is taken in 2–4 divided doses daily beginning the day before traveling and continuing until 2 days after returning home from trips."

As to other natural medicines for TD, the CDC says, "The use of probiotics, such as *Lactobacillus GG* and *Saccharomyces boulardii*, has been studied in the prevention of TD in small numbers of people. Results are inconclusive, partially because standardized preparations of these bacteria are not reliably available. Studies are ongoing with probiotics to prevent TD, but data are insufficient to recommend their use. There have been anecdotal reports of beneficial outcomes after using bovine colostrum as a daily prophylaxis agent for TD; however, because no data from rigorous clinical trials demonstrate efficacy, there is insufficient information to recommend the use of bovine colostrum to prevent TD."[9]

Nevertheless, ConsumerLab.com advises, "The specific strains in the probiotics *Culturelle®* and *Florastor®* have been shown to help prevent traveler's diarrhea, with *Culturelle®* being the least expensive. . . . For travel, start a few days before travel and continue during travel." I'll discuss their prices in the next section.

Antibiotic-Associated Diarrhea

In my practice in Colorado Springs, we're finding increasing interest among patients for preventing antibiotic-associated diarrhea. However, among available products, there is a wide variation in dosing depending on the particular probiotic strain.

Harvard Health says, "The best case for probiotic therapy has been in the treatment of antibiotic-associated diarrhea," adding, "Two large reviews, taken together, suggest that probiotics reduce antibiotic-associated diarrhea by 60 percent when compared with a placebo."[10]

Natural Medicines advises, "*Saccharomyces boulardii* 250–500 mg two to four times a day, usually not to exceed 1000 mg daily, has been most commonly used during antibiotic treatment. A specific strain *Lactobacillus GG* is the most well-studied lactobacillus product for this use. Dosing used in clinical research include 6–40 billion colony-forming units of *Lactobacillus GG* daily. In most cases, lactobacillus treatment is initiated within two days of starting antibiotic treatment and continued for at least three days after antibiotic treatment." *Natural Medicines* lists both as "Likely Safe" and "Possibly Effective."

To prevent antibiotic-associated diarrhea, *Natural Medicines* says, "Clinical research shows that patients who take a probiotic along with an antibiotic often have a reduction in the risk of antibiotic-associated diarrhea. The magnitude of this effect depends on the specific probiotic or strain used. Overall, clinical research shows that taking a lactobacillus-containing probiotic reduces the risk of antibiotic-associated diarrhea by about 36 to 70 percent, while taking *Saccharomyces boulardii* can decrease the risk of antibiotic-associated diarrhea by 52 to 63 percent." Therefore, *Natural Medicines* rates *Saccharomyces boulardii* (i.e., *Florastor®*) as "Likely Effective" and lactobacillus-containing probiotics (i.e., *Culturelle®* and others) as "Possibly Effective."

Natural Medicines adds, "Bifidobacterium species are also commonly included in probiotic products used for antibiotic-associated diarrhea, but clinical research is inconsistent. A variety of combination probiotic products have also been studied for this use . . . with reductions of about 34 to 48 percent; however, not all research supports the use of probiotic combinations." They consider this "Insufficient Evidence" to recommend bifidobacterium products for this indication, adding, "As is the case with infectious and travelers' diarrhea, evidence on the use of milk or yogurt fermented with various probiotic strains is mixed."

The 2020 AGA clinical guidelines concluded that the overall quality of the evidence was rated as "Low," adding, "the analysis of most studies [included] the potential for some benefit, as well as for some harm." In addition, "It should be pointed out that beneficial effect of probiotics was seen mainly in patients with very high risk of developing [antibiotic-associated diarrhea]. . . . Thus, patients who place a high value on avoiding associated financial cost or potential harms (especially those immunocompromised patients) and who have low risk of developing [antibiotic-associated diarrhea] (mainly outpatients in the community) may choose not to use any probiotics."[11]

In 2020, ConsumerLab's "Top Picks" for preventing antibiotic-associated diarrhea were *Culturelle® Probiotics Digestive Health* (*Lactobacillus GG*, 37 cents per vegetarian capsule containing 10 billion cells) and, at a much higher cost, *FloraStor®* (*Saccharomyces boulardii lyo* CNCM 1–745, $1.94 for two vegetable capsules containing a total of 6 billion cells).

ConsumerLab adds, "Either should be started the same day as when starting antibiotic treatment and continued for one week after finishing the antibiotic. Take the probiotic at least two hours after the antibiotic." In late 2020, I was able to find *Culturelle®* with 10 billion CFUs per capsule online for about 30 cents and *Culturelle®* with 15 billion CFUs for about 67 cents per capsule. *Florastor®* was $1.22 per two capsules.

Florastor® is NMBER® rated 9 out of 10 while *Culturelle®* is rated 8 out of 10. If cost is not an issue, I recommend *Florastor®* first and *Culturelle®* second as options for my patients to consider when I prescribe an antibiotic.

Constipation

Constipation is one of the most common GI problems in the US. The most common definition is when you have fewer than three bowel movements a week. However, it can also include other symptoms such as hard stools, having to strain to have a bowel movement, or having a sense of incomplete evacuation afterward. Chronic constipation is when these symptoms last for several weeks or longer.[12] It is ubiquitous, with 16 percent of American adults suffering from chronic constipation and one in four having it at least once a year. The number of people seen by doctors for this has more than doubled in the last two decades, even though most people handle it on their own, resulting in national spending on over-the-counter laxatives running into the billions of dollars each year. It's been called "an American epidemic."[13] To prevent it, the Cleveland Clinic advises several steps:

- eat a well-balanced diet with plenty of fiber
- stay hydrated (drink water)
- exercise regularly
- move your bowels when you feel the urge (do not wait)
- treat mild constipation with a dietary supplement[14]

While psyllium and prunes are proven treatments for chronic constipation, Asian studies have suggested that fresh kiwi may also reduce symptoms. A wide variety of over-the-counter treatments includes

- bulk-forming laxatives such as methylcellulose (*Citrucel®*) and psyllium hydrophilic mucilloid (*Metamucil®*),
- stool softeners such as *Colace®* and *Surfak®*,
- stimulant laxatives (which are the fastest acting) such as aloe, cascara, senna compounds (*Ex-Lax®*, *Senokot®*), bisacodyl (*Dulco-lax®*, *Correctol®*), and castor oil,
- laxatives such as milk of magnesia and magnesium citrate, and
- osmotic-type laxatives such as *MiraLax®*.[15]

The popularity of probiotics for treating constipation in adults is growing rapidly. *Natural Medicines* writes, "A meta-analysis of clinical research in adults with functional constipation shows that taking probiotics increases the number of bowel movements by about 1.3 movements per week when compared with placebo. One specific probiotic species, *Lactobacillus reuteri* DSM 17938 (*BioGaia*® *Chewable Tablets*, NMBER rated 8 out of 10), has the best evidence of benefit." I was able to find *BioGaia*® for about 88 cents per chewable tablet.

Natural Medicines adds, "Other single-strain or combination probiotic products containing lactobacillus and/or bifidobacteria species have also shown benefit in clinical research [e.g., *HEXBIO*® *by B-Crobes*, NMBER rated 8 out of 10]." *Natural Medicines* concludes, "Overall, the evidence for the use of probiotics for reducing symptoms of constipation is promising. However, because most of the available studies evaluate different probiotic strains, additional research is needed to confirm which strains might be most beneficial."

For treating constipation in adults, ConsumerLab's "Top Pick" is "*Gerber Soothe*® *Probiotic Colic Drops* (containing *Lactobacillus reuteri* DSM 17938). Although a relatively small amount of cells, 5 drops (providing 100 million cells and costing 40 cents) given twice daily has been shown to reduce constipation in adults."

Indigestion and Dyspepsia (Gastrointestinal Reflux Disease [GERD] or Heartburn)

The umbrella term *dyspepsia* or *indigestion* in the stomach area of your upper abdomen (epigastric region) refers to a pervasive problem experienced by about 30 percent of the US population in any year.[16] It consists of intermittent or recurrent discomfort, burning, or pain in the upper abdomen, early fullness while eating a meal, bloating of the stomach, nausea, or feeling uncomfortably full after eating a meal. About one-third of the time, it can be a sign of an underlying serious problem such as an ulcer, stomach cancer, or a common stomach infection with *Helicobacter pylori* (*H pylori*) bacteria.

Three of the more common causes of dyspepsia are acid reflux, heartburn, and gastroesophageal reflux disease (GERD). These terms are erroneously used interchangeably.[17]

Acid reflux is the general term for a prevalent problem that can range from mild to severe and occurs when the digestive acids made in the stomach flow back (reflux) into the lower part of the tube connecting the mouth and stomach (the esophagus). This backwash (acid reflux) can irritate the lining of the esophagus.[18]

Despite its name, *heartburn*, which is usually caused by acid reflux, has nothing to do with the heart. The name derives from the fact that some of the symptoms mimic those of a heart attack. *GERD* is the chronic, more severe form of acid reflux. Most adults have heartburn once in a while; however, about 20 percent have it at least once a week. GERD is either (1) mild acid reflux that occurs at least twice a week or (2) moderate to severe acid reflux that occurs at least once a week. Most people can manage the discomfort of GERD with lifestyle changes and over-the-counter medications. But some people with GERD may need more potent drugs or surgery to ease symptoms.[19]

Untreated GERD can lead to long-term problems such as esophagitis, ulcers, or scarring or chronic changes in the lining of the esophagus called *Barrett's esophagus*, which increases the likelihood of cancer of the esophagus. Fortunately, only a small percentage of people with GERD develop Barrett's esophagus.[20] Nevertheless, before treating dyspepsia with prescription drugs, over-the-counter remedies, or natural medicines, a 2020 review recommended the following:[21]

1. Endoscopy should be performed for all patients sixty years and older with at least one month of dyspepsia symptoms.

2. For patients younger than sixty years, an *H pylori* test should be done first. If negative, then treatment of excess stomach acid is appropriate.

3. All patients should be advised to limit foods associated with increased symptoms of dyspepsia; a diet low in FODMAPs is suggested (Healthline has a good article, "FODMAP 101: A Detailed Beginner's Guide," at tinyurl.com/y8wghdod).

4. Along with these three recommendations, an eight-week trial of acid suppression therapy is recommended.

5. If acid suppression does not alleviate symptoms, patients should be treated with tricyclic antidepressants (we know a low-dose

tricyclic can improve the symptoms of dyspepsia, particularly epigastric pain, but just how it does so is not clear) followed by prokinetics (medications that help control acid reflux) and psychological therapy (as it has been shown that psychological treatment techniques can help ease GI distress or at least help a person cope much better with their GI symptoms). The routine use of complementary and alternative medicine therapies has not shown evidence of effectiveness and is not recommended.

If the *H pylori* test for those younger than sixty comes back normal, which it does 70 percent of the time when no disease is found, then the condition is called *functional dyspepsia*.[22]

In addition, "Complementary and alternative therapies are not recommended by the ACG/CAG [American College of Gastroenterology/ Canadian Association of Gastroenterology] dyspepsia guidelines, although it is accepted that patients may wish to try them, particularly if conventional treatments have proven ineffective. Nevertheless, it is important to emphasize that there is currently no clear evidence to support their use."[23]

However, there may be at least three reasons people are choosing natural medicines instead of prescription or over-the-counter medications for indigestion or dyspepsia.

First, among the top medical stories in 2019 was the discovery of contaminants in ranitidine—best known as *Zantac®*. It was a "probable human carcinogen" (cancer-causing) substance known as *NDMA*. In April 2020, the FDA requested that manufacturers pull all prescription and over-the-counter ranitidine drugs from the market immediately. The FDA noted that an ongoing investigation determined levels of NDMA increased over time and when stored at higher-than-normal temperatures, thus posing an immediate risk to public health.[24] The FDA also reported the recall of several lots of nizatidine (*Axid®*), a similar drug, again because of NDMA. The FDA said the recalls "are a new cause for alarm for the 15 million Americans who take ranitidine at prescription levels, and the millions more who regularly take lower-dose, over-the-counter versions" as "*Zantac®* was once the best-selling drug in the world."[25]

Second, there are two nutrient depletion issues of which you need to be aware with two forms of drugs that reduce gastric acid in the stomach:

1. The "H2 blockers," which include cimetidine (*Tagamet®, Tagamet HB®*), famotidine (*Pepcid®, Pepcid AC®*), nizatidine (*Axid®*), ranitidine (*Zantac®*), all have a moderate risk of causing depletion of vitamin B12.

2. The Proton Pump Inhibitors (PPIs), the more common of which include omeprazole (*Prilosec®, Prilosec OTC®*), lansoprazole (*Prevacid®, Prevacid 24-Hour®*), rabeprazole (*Aciphex®, Aciphex Sprinkle®*), pantoprazole (*Protonix®*), esomeprazole (*Nexium®, Nexium 24 HR®*), all have a moderate risk of causing depletion of vitamin B12 and a major risk of causing depletion of magnesium.

Third, long-term use of PPIs has been associated with a low risk of kidney and heart disease, stomach cancer, type 2 diabetes, as well as fractures, pneumonia, and dementia.[26]

As more people learn of these potential difficulties, they may consider looking at natural medicines for indigestion or dyspepsia. To that end, *Natural Medicines* rates two substances as "Effective" and "Possibly Safe": calcium carbonate and magnesium. They rate one as "Possibly Effective" and "Possibly Safe": phosphate salts.

CALCIUM CARBONATE is the natural medication I most commonly recommend for dyspepsia. *Natural Medicines* says "Taking calcium carbonate orally as an antacid is effective for treating dyspepsia (specifically calcium carbonate in doses of 500 to 1000 mg a day). Calcium carbonate has FDA approval as an antacid." They also judge it "Likely Safe" when used short-term. In general, taking calcium carbonate before a meal provides about a half hour of relief. However, *Natural Medicines* warns health professionals, "Calcium can . . . prevent absorption of many drugs . . . including levothyroxine (and others). . . . Advise patients to take these drugs either two hours before or six hours after taking calcium supplements." Some well-known calcium carbonate products, all FDA approved as OTC products and NMBER rated 9 out of 10, include *Caltrate®, Os-Cal®*, and *Tums®*. Chew the tablets well before swallowing for faster relief. Of course, you'll want to choose one with a flavor you like.

MAGNESIUM. *Natural Medicines* states, "Taking magnesium orally as an antacid reduces symptoms of gastric hyperacidity or GERD. Typically, magnesium carbonate, hydroxide, oxide, or trisilicate salts are used. Magnesium hydroxide has the fastest onset of action. Magnesium carbonate is slower due to its crystal structure. Magnesium trisilicate has the slowest onset and longest duration due to poor solubility." They add, "Orally, magnesium can cause gastrointestinal irritation, nausea, vomiting, and diarrhea." Because of magnesium's laxative effect, the most common side effect is diarrhea. Also, magnesium products should not be used by patients with kidney problems. Finally, magnesium, like calcium, has the potential to attach to some drugs and render them insoluble and unabsorbable. It's another reason we recommend checking with your physician or pharmacist before taking a natural medicine with prescription or over-the-counter medications. You can also use a web-based interaction checker. Drugs.com has a nice one at tinyurl.com/zq7bqxj.

PHOSPHATE SALTS. Aluminum phosphate and calcium phosphate are FDA-permitted ingredients of over-the-counter antacids. But calcium carbonate is more likely to be effective and less likely to cause side effects, particularly loose stools.

Quite a number of other natural medicines, including many herbs, have been evaluated for dyspepsia, but they are either only "Possibly Effective" or have "Insufficient Evidence" for safety or effectiveness. I've indicated them in the following chart. In addition, ACG/CAG says, "Acupuncture has also been investigated for the treatment of FD [functional dyspepsia]. However, good quality trials are lacking, and a Cochrane review concluded that there was insufficient evidence to be able to draw firm conclusions on its efficacy. Chinese herbal remedies may be effective for treating FD . . . but most studies are small, with a high risk of bias, . . . meaning further rigorous studies are needed. Similarly, there is little evidence for the use of either probiotics or homeopathy in dyspepsia."[27]

In the following charts, I have included the evaluation by *Natural Medicines* of the most commonly used natural medicines. Where data is available, I'll differentiate short-term versus long-term use. In addition, for probiotics, because of long names and complex ingredients, I'll often use brand names. More detailed information is available from ConsumerLab .com and *Natural Medicines*.

Natural Medicines for Infectious Diarrhea (ID), including Rotavirus Diarrhea (RVD) and Traveler's Diarrhea (TD)

Safety / Effective	Likely Safe	Possibly Safe
Effective	★★★★★	★★★
Likely Effective	★★★★ • Bismuth (TD – short term) • Probiotics such as Culturelle and others that contain Lactobacillus GG (ID, RVD) • Saccharomyces boulardii (ID, RVD)	★★
Possibly Effective	★★★ • Banana • Bifidobacteria (RVD, TD) • Blond psyllium • Bovine colostrum (RVD) • Carob • Fermented milk (RVD) • Guar gum • Lactobacillus (TD) • Massage • Probiotic • Florastor (RVD, TD) • Saccharomyces boulardii (TD) • Sangre de Grado (TD) • Soy	★ • Clay (short term) • Fermented milk • German chamomile
Insufficient evidence for safety or effectiveness AND/OR evidence for lack of safety or effectiveness		
☹ • Apple • Bacillus coagulans • Berberine • Black tea • Carrot • Casein protein • Coconut oil • Copper • Docosahexaenoic acid (DHA) • Folic acid (vitamin B9) • Fructo-oligosaccharides (FOS) (TD)	• Glutamine • Homeopathic products • Honey • Hyperimmune egg (RVD) • Moxibustion • Omega-6 fatty acids • Pectin • Tormentil (RVD) • Vitamin B12 (cobalamin) • White pepper • Yogurt	

Natural Medicines for Antibiotic-Associated Diarrhea

Safety Effective	Likely Safe	Possibly Safe
Likely Effective	★★★★ • Probiotics containing Saccharomyces boulardii • Florastor	★★★

Possibly
Effective
	★★★
	• Probiotics containing lactobacillus
	  • Actimel
	  • BioGaia
	  • Bio-K+ Cl1285
	  • Culturelle
	  • DanActive
	  • Florajen
	  • ProViva
		★★
		• Fermented milk

Insufficient evidence for safety or effectiveness AND/OR evidence for lack of safety or effectiveness

• Bifidobacteria
• Inulin
• Kefir
• Probiotics
  • AB Yogurt
  • Ecologic AAD
  • Lactinex
• Yogurt

Natural Medicines for Constipation

Safety / Effective	Likely Safe	Possibly Safe
Effective	★★★★★ • Black psyllium • Blond psyllium • Kiwi • Magnesium • Prunes	★★★
Likely Effective	★★★★ • Phosphate salts (short term) • Senna (short term) – FDA-approved non-prescription drug	★★ • European buckthorn (short term) • Glycerol (short term)

Possibly Effective	★★★
	• Bifidobacteria
	• Biofeedback
	• Castor bean (short term)
	• Guar gum
	• Karaya gum
	• Lactobacillus
	• Olive
	• Plum
	• Probiotics
	  • BioGaia chewables
	  • Hexbio
	• Wheat bran
	• Xanthan gum
	• Yogurt
		★
		• Alder buckthorn (short term)
		• Aloe (short term)
		• Cascara sagrada (short term)
		• Elderberry
		• Elderflower (short term)
		• Fructo-oligosaccharides (FOS)
		• Glucomannan powder
		• Inulin (short term)

Insufficient evidence for safety or effectiveness AND/OR evidence for lack of safety or effectiveness		
☹ • Acupuncture • Alder buckthorn (long term) • Anise • Cascara sagrada (long term) • Castor bean (long term) • Cocoa • Coriander • Corydalis • Cupping • Fennel • Fermented milk • Flaxseed, ground	• Galacto-oligosaccharides (GOS) • Hemp seed • Kefir • Mallow • Massage • Moxibustion • Pantothenic acid • Polydextrose • Probiotics, in general • Rye grass • Senna (long term) • Zizyphus	

Natural Medicines for Dyspepsia, Heartburn, and Gastroesophageal Reflux Disease (GERD)

Safe / Effective	Likely Safe	Possibly Safe
Effective	★★★★★ • Calcium carbonate or citrate • Magnesium	★★★
Likely Effective	★★★★ • Phosphate salts	★★
Possibly Effective	★★★ • Angelica • Milk thistle • Peppermint oil	★ • Anise • Artichoke • Caraway • Clown's mustard plant (short term) • German chamomile (short term) • Indian gooseberry (GERD) • Lemon balm • Licorice (short term) • Mastic

Insufficient evidence for safety or effectiveness AND/OR evidence for lack of safety or effectiveness

☹ • Activated charcoal (short term) • Acupuncture • Astaxanthin • Betaine anhydrous (GERD) • Bitter orange • Black seed • Blond psyllium (GERD) • Capsicum • Casein protein (GERD) • Chinese herbal remedies • Chondroitin sulfate (GERD) • Corydalis (GERD) • Fenugreek (GERD) • Ginger	• Greater celandine • Hyaluronic acid (GERD) • Homeopathic products • Iberogast • Massage (GERD) • Melatonin (GERD) • Myrtle (GERD) • Pectin (GERD) • Perilla • Probiotics • Quince (GERD) • Rikkunshito • Sea buckthorn • Turmeric

The recommendations in the charts are based almost entirely on the "Safety and Effectiveness Ratings" contained in *Natural Medicines™* and explained in chapter 4 of this book. They assume the use of high-quality, uncontaminated products and the use of typical doses. Keep in mind that some products are never appropriate for some patients due to concomitant disease states, potential drug interactions, or other clinical factors. Details are available at *Natural Medicines™*.

13

Healthy Hair and Hair Loss

According to the American Hair Loss Association, "American hair loss sufferers spend more than $3.5 billion a year in an attempt to treat their hair loss [as much as is spent for over-the-counter cold and flu treatments]. Unfortunately, 99 percent of all products being marketed in the less than ethical hair loss treatment industry are completely ineffective for the majority of those who use them." As a result, the Association recommends "against purchasing any hair loss product that is not approved by the FDA or recommended by the American Hair Loss Association."[1]

The American Academy of Dermatology (AAD) recommends that hair loss should first be evaluated by your family physician or a dermatologist (specialists who treat the skin, hair, and nails). These physicians have the expertise and tools to help them "get to the root cause" (pun intended) of your hair loss—which could come from any number of medical, skin, hair, or even emotional disorders. The reason to see a doctor early, as opposed to treating it on your own, is that the sooner you find the cause, the better your outcome. In other words, the less hair you have lost, the more successful legitimate treatments tend to be. Early treatment is by far the most effective.[2]

The Huffington Post points out, "Hair loss, common for men and many women in midlife, can have profound emotional and psychological effects. . . . The phenomenon can be particularly devastating for [women].

'With men, hair loss in midlife is expected, and they can still be seen as attractive,' says [Spencer] Kobren, [founder and president of the American Hair Loss Association], 'But for a woman, it is over.' This makes women especially vulnerable to all manner of hair loss 'cures,' and the possibility of spending lots of money, time, and emotional investment on ineffective treatments."[3]

There are two common forms of hair loss: hereditary baldness and diffuse hair loss.

Androgenic Alopecia (Hereditary Baldness)

In 2019, *Prevention Magazine* estimated that 80 million US adults experienced the most common type of hair loss, androgenic alopecia.[4] It used to be called *male-pattern baldness* but is now called *hereditary baldness* as it affects an estimated 30 million women in the US.[5] According to Mayo Clinic, the safest and most effective pharmaceutical medications to combat this type of hair loss are minoxidil and finasteride.[6]

MINOXIDIL (*Rogaine®*) is an over-the-counter medication approved for men and women. It is rubbed into the scalp daily and is available in 2 percent and 5 percent liquid or foam. The 5 percent products are most often marketed to men, although women may safely use them as well. I recommend the 5 percent foam for two reasons: studies show that the 5 percent products are more effective and that the foam formulations are free of propylene glycol, which can cause skin irritation.[7] Robert Griffith, MD, of Alabama Dermatology Associates, advises, "There is also a small increased risk of irritation from the higher concentration, but most patients tolerate it well. At least six months of treatment is required to prevent further hair loss and to start hair regrowth. Only a small percentage of patients obtain clinically significant new growth, but the majority attain maintenance of their hair, which is an improvement as the condition is slowly progressive without any treatment." It must be used indefinitely for continued support of existing hair follicles and the maintenance of any experienced hair regrowth.

FINASTERIDE (*Propecia®*, *Proscar®*) is a prescription drug approved for men that is taken as a pill. Over the first two years of use, up to 90 percent of men taking it experience a slowing of hair loss and improvement in hair thickening. About two-thirds show some new hair growth.[8] It must also be used indefinitely and may not work as well for men over sixty years old.

Finasteride comes in 1 mg and 5 mg tablets. Multiple studies show the 1 mg dose is just as effective as 5 mg. Although higher-quality studies are needed, small trials suggest that finasteride may be more effective than minoxidil for the induction of hair growth. In addition, one small study suggested that combination therapy with finasteride and topical minoxidil may be superior to monotherapy with either agent; further study is needed to determine whether combination therapy should be routinely recommended.

However, the effect of finasteride on prostate cancer screening and sexual functioning should be discussed with your family physician. The FDA warns that pregnant women should not take it or even handle crushed or broken pills due to risk to their unborn baby.

Natural Medicines for Hereditary Baldness

In animal studies, pumpkin seed oil (PSO) has been shown to increase hair growth. *Natural Medicines*™ rates PSO as "Possibly Effective" and "Possibly Safe" in treating hereditary baldness "based upon a study from South Korea which suggested taking a particular pumpkin seed oil (*Octa Sabal Plus*, Dreamplus Co. Ltd.). 400 mg daily in divided doses for 24 weeks increased hair count by 30 percent compared to placebo in men with mild to moderate hair loss. Self-rated improvement and satisfaction scores were 62 percent and 52 percent higher with PSO vs. placebo, respectively."

Dr. Worthington reminds us, "Our 'Possibly Effective' rating does not mean that we would recommend these products, but that this product has some clinical evidence supporting its use for a specific indication; however, the evidence is limited by quantity, quality, or contradictory findings. These products might be beneficial but do not have enough high-quality evidence to recommend for most people."

This product is not available in the US but may be available online (with all the associated risks of ordering natural medicines online). In addition, *Octa Sabal Plus* contained a variety of other ingredients that may stimulate hair growth, such as evening primrose oil and red clover—so there's no way to know whether the PSO or the combination is what worked.

However, no PSO products are NMBER® rated greater than 7 out of 10 nor are any PSO products rated by ConsumerLab.com, Labdoor, or USP®.

According to ConsumerLab, "There is some very preliminary evidence that saw palmetto extract and beta-sitosterol may be beneficial in androgenic alopecia (hereditary baldness)—possibly by inhibiting the same enzyme (5-alpha-reductase) inhibited by the finasteride." *Natural Medicines* cautions, "The effects of saw palmetto when taken orally by patients with androgenic alopecia are inconsistent and unclear," and "taking saw palmetto extract 320 mg daily for 24 months is less effective at improving hair growth in men with androgenic alopecia compared to taking finasteride 1 [one] mg daily."

Natural Medicines also discusses the clinical research on "a combination of saw palmetto extract 200 mg plus beta-sitosterol 50 mg taken twice daily." They report that this "improves subjective scores of hair quantity and quality in men with androgenic alopecia" and "some early clinical research shows that saw palmetto lotion applied topically twice daily for 50 weeks improves hair density by 27 percent in men and women with androgenic alopecia."

However, an improvement of 13 percent was observed in the placebo group, and no between-group comparisons were made. Therefore, it is unclear if saw palmetto provided a statistically significant improvement compared to placebo." *Natural Medicines* rates saw palmetto and beta-sitosterol as having "Insufficient Evidence" to rate for hereditary baldness.

Alopecia Areata and Diffuse Hair Loss

Alopecia areata is an autoimmune disease that most commonly leads to focal patches of hair loss. Diffuse hair loss that is not caused by an autoimmune disease is a far more common form of hair loss in women and may be improved by the application of OTC minoxidil. Although minoxidil is not yet approved by the FDA for this problem, MedScape writes, "In those with extensive disease (50–99 percent hair loss), response rates vary from eight to forty-five percent."[9]

A number of other treatments are available from a dermatologist, although most generally have limited effectiveness. However, dermatologic breakthroughs are occurring quite often as our knowledge of hair loss expands. Your local dermatologist or family physician is the best information source for new research.

In the meantime, in the natural medicines' realm, certain essential oils are sold to apply directly to the scalp. *Natural Medicines* rates two substances as "Possibly Safe" but with "insufficient reliable evidence to rate" for effectiveness when used topically in treating alopecia areata: Atlantic cedar and lavender. They write, "There is some evidence that topically applying lavender oil in combination with the essential oils from thyme, rosemary, and Atlantic cedar (cedarwood) improves hair growth in up to 44 percent of patients after seven months of treatment." You can find the recipe and technique at tinyurl.com/tk9oe3r.

Other Natural Medicines for Hair Growth

A number of other natural medicines are promoted for hair growth, including biotin (vitamin B7), coenzyme Q10, garlic, L-carnitine, raspberry ketone, red clover, rosemary, and thyme. *Natural Medicines* says there is "Insufficient Evidence" to rate any of these for hereditary baldness or alopecia areata.

ConsumerLab adds, "Cysteine and acetyl-cysteine supplements have been promoted for hair growth (typically 500 mg daily), although evidence for this use is not conclusive." In addition, "Biotin is often included as an ingredient in supplements for hair and nails, but there is little evidence that it is helpful for hair loss." They add, "A symptom of biotin deficiency is hair loss—although taking biotin if you are not deficient won't help your hair."

Medications That May Cause Hair Loss

To make a complex issue even more complicated, it's important to know that a number of natural medicines are associated with the side effect of hair loss, including DHEA, selenium, St. John's wort, vitamin A, and zinc. Also, there are a number of prescription medications that may lead to hair loss, including drugs used to treat gout, arthritis, depression, high blood pressure, and heart problems. Even the birth control pill has been linked to hair loss in some women.

The Bottom Line

When it comes to natural medicines and hair loss, I can't recommend any of them as being both "Safe" and "Effective." Furthermore, the traditional medications most often recommended are generally safe, somewhat effective, and reasonably priced. Generic prescription finasteride, for example, for men can often be purchased for under $10 per month (in some areas it's as low as $3 per month), which is far less than any of these natural medicines. The OTC topical medication, minoxidil, used for men and women can be found for under $15 per month.

Even though I do not have the space to discuss many other natural medicines pushed for these indications, I've included the ratings for some of the more common ones in the following charts. More detailed information is available from ConsumerLab.com and *Natural Medicines*.

Prescription and Natural Medicines for Hair Loss
(Androgenic Alopecia or Hereditary Baldness)

Safe / Effective	Likely Safe	Possibly Safe
Effective	★★★★★	★★
Likely Effective	★★★★ • finasteride (Propecia) • minoxidil (Rogaine)	★★
Possibly Effective	★★★	★ • Pumpkin seed oil (topical)
Insufficient evidence for safety or effectiveness AND/OR evidence for lack of safety or effectiveness		
☹ • Apple or apple polyphenols (topical) • Beta-sitosterol • Mineral supplements		• Multivitamins • Onion juice (topical) • Raspberry ketone (topical) • Saw palmetto extract

Prescriptions and Natural Medicines for Hair Loss
(Alopecia Areata and Diffuse Hair Loss)

Safe / Effective	Likely Safe	Possibly Safe
Effective	★★★★★	★★
Likely Effective	★★★★ • minoxidil (Rogaine)	★★
Possibly Effective	★★★	★ • Essential oils of Atlantic cedar, lavender, rosemary, and thyme (topical)
Insufficient evidence for safety or effectiveness AND/OR evidence for lack of safety or effectiveness		
⊗ • Atlantic cedar oil (topical) • Biotin (vitamin B7) • Coenzyme Q10 • Cysteine • Garlic • Lavender oil (topical)	• L-carnitine • Mineral supplements • Multivitamins • Raspberry ketone (topical) • Red clover (topical) • Rosemary (topical) • Thyme (topical)	

Most of the recommendations in the charts are based on the "Safety and Effectiveness Ratings" contained in *Natural Medicines*™ and explained in chapter 4 of this book. They assume the use of high-quality, uncontaminated products and the use of typical doses. Keep in mind that some products are never appropriate for some patients due to concomitant disease states, potential drug interactions, or other clinical factors. Details are available at *Natural Medicines*™.

14

Heart Health, Hypertension, and Heart Attack

The American Heart Association (AHA) reports that cardiovascular disease (CVD) is the leading cause of death for men and women as well as virtually all racial and ethnic groups in the US. About every forty seconds in America, one person has a heart attack and another has a stroke. The 850,000 who die from CVD each year represent one in every four deaths in the US, costing about 351 billion USD each year.[1]

In 2017, nearly half a million deaths in the US included hypertension as a primary or contributing cause.[2] The AMA says, "High blood pressure is the nation's leading risk factor for heart attack and stroke, yet an overwhelming number of US adults are living with uncontrolled high blood pressure."[3] The CDC points out, "Half of adults (30 million) with blood pressure ≥140/90 mm Hg who should be taking medication to control their blood pressure aren't prescribed or aren't taking medication."[4]

Researchers at the Barbra Streisand Women's Heart Center at Cedars-Sinai Medical Center in Los Angeles reported that among adult women in the US, less than half are aware that CVD is the leading threat to women's lives. Most thought breast cancer posed a more significant risk. They are wrong.[5] AHA's "Go Red for Women" points out, "While 1 in 31 American women dies from breast cancer each year, 1 in 3 dies of heart disease. Heart disease and stroke cause 1 in 3 deaths among women each year—more than all cancers combined."[6]

To put this in perspective, the CDC tells us that each year in America, about 40,000 women die from breast cancer, while more than ten times that number (~425,000) die from CVD.[7] "Since 1984, more women than men have died each year from heart disease, and the gap between men and women's survival continues to widen," adds Go Red for Women. "Fortunately, we can change that because 80 percent of cardiac and stroke events may be prevented with education and action."[8]

No wonder so many people are interested in natural medicines for heart health. Unfortunately, most are looking for heart health in all the wrong places—trying to replace proven lifestyle changes with ineffective, expensive, and potentially dangerous supplements. I'm surprised that only 28 percent of people ages fifty-five years or older take natural medicines for heart health daily.[9] Nevertheless, this still represents about 34 percent of the US population or about 100 million Americans that may be wasting their hard-earned money.

Given the conflicting studies and endless advertising over the last few decades, I must confess I was one of them. I have a strong family history of heart disease, heart attack, high lipids, and diabetes, and I have at various times taken and recommended multiple supplements over the last three decades. But for the last several years, I have not taken *any* supplements for heart health or to prevent heart disease. Why? Simply put, there's no longer reliable evidence for their safety and efficacy.

Choosing Wisely (an initiative that seeks to advance a national dialogue on avoiding unnecessary medical tests, treatments, and procedures) adds, "These products [supplements] are heavily marketed. For many years, people believed claims that they could help prevent heart disease and cancer. There has now been a great deal of research on these claims. And the research shows that most people don't benefit from taking supplements. And some supplements can be harmful for some people."[10]

Before we examine the natural medicines touted for heart health, let's review some basics—and this is the most important takeaway from this chapter. Monique Tello, MD, MPH, a contributing editor for *Harvard Health*, writes,[11]

What if I could prescribe a pill that could prevent or treat high blood pressure, diabetes, high cholesterol, heart disease, even depression and dementia? And what if researchers had extensively researched this pill and the result was: ample proof that it's effective. On top of that, it's practically free and has no bad side effects. As a matter of fact, its only side effects are improved sleep, increased energy, and weight loss.

Actually, folks, this powerful medicine exists. It's real and readily available for everyone. It's called *intensive lifestyle change*. Its active ingredients are physical activity and drastic improvements in diet, and it works well. Amazingly well. If it were an actual pill, no doubt millions of people would be clamoring for it, and some pharmaceutical company would reap massive profits. But here's how you can get "it." Intensive lifestyle changes involve knowledge and action.

She bases her recommendations on scores of studies that have examined modifiable risk factors for CVD. Nonmodifiable factors include things such as family history, ethnicity, and age. But there are plenty of things that can be modified, and the impact can be massive.

The CDC explains, "High blood pressure, high blood cholesterol, and smoking are key risk factors for heart disease. About half of Americans (47 percent) have at least one of these three risk factors." They add, "Several other medical conditions and lifestyle choices can also put people at a higher risk for heart disease, including diabetes, overweight and obesity, unhealthy diet, physical inactivity, and excessive alcohol use."[12]

Each of these is modifiable—in other words, highly treatable with lifestyle changes that are *far* more effective than *any* natural medicine. Let's start with the "knowledge" piece of Dr. Tello's advice. There are five numbers you should be aware of (knowledge) and five lifestyle habits you should practice (action) for improved heart health.

The ABCDEs of Heart Health

If you don't know your five numbers, you risk putting the quality and quantity of your life on the line. I tell my patients: you need to know your ABCDEs:

1. **A = A1C.** According to the NIH, one-third of people with diabetes (elevated levels of blood sugar or glucose) don't know they have

it.[13] Even worse, almost 90 percent of adults with prediabetes are undiagnosed. An estimated 34 percent of US adults have prediabetes, and this rises to nearly half of adults age sixty-five years or older.[14] Untreated prediabetes or diabetes leads to many severe problems, including CVD, kidney disease, and premature death. A blood test called *glycohemoglobin* or *A1C* can tell you your average blood sugar level for the previous three months and is used to diagnose prediabetes and diabetes. The American Diabetes Association (ADA) recommends regular screening for diabetes starting at age forty-five (using either a blood glucose test or an A1C), with repeated tests at least every three years.[15] The USPSTF recommends screening for abnormal blood glucose as part of cardiovascular risk assessment in adults ages forty to seventy years who are overweight or obese;[16] however, this represents about 70 percent of all adults.[17]

2. **B = BMI.** Body mass index (BMI) is a useful measure of overweight and obesity. It is calculated from your height and weight and estimates your body fat. It is a reasonably good gauge of your risk for diseases such as heart disease, high blood pressure, type 2 diabetes, stroke, and certain cancers.[18] Although BMI can be used for most people, it does have some limits: it may overestimate body fat in athletes and others who have a muscular build, and it may underestimate body fat in older persons and others who have lost muscle. There are many BMI calculators on the internet. A good one can be found at tinyurl.com/qyqhmdx.

3. **C = Cholesterol.** The AHA recommends a lipoprotein profile be taken every four to six years, starting at age twenty. This is a blood test that calculates your total cholesterol, healthy (HDL) cholesterol, lethal (LDL) cholesterol, and triglycerides (TG).[19] You may need to be tested more frequently or have more advanced tests if your physician determines that you have an increased risk for heart disease or stroke. The USPSTF recommends lipid testing in all adults ages forty to seventy-five years.[20]

4. **D = Diastolic and systolic blood pressures.** The AHA recommends that all adults twenty or older get their blood pressure (BP) checked at least once every two years as long as it is below 120/80

mm mercury (Hg).[21] The upper number is the *systolic blood pressure*, and the lower number is the *diastolic blood pressure*. The USPSTF recommends screening for high blood pressure starting at eighteen years of age. Both the AHA and USPSTF recommend that people with high blood pressure obtain BP readings away from the doctor's office—for example, with home BP monitoring—before starting treatment. This is a crucial recommendation because BP readings from an ambulatory BP device are more predictive of adverse outcomes and even all-cause mortality. Why? Merely going to a medical facility can raise the BP of many people.[22] In fact, ambulatory systolic BP tends to average nineteen points lower, while diastolic BP averages eleven points lower than when measured in the medical office setting.[23] If your systolic is 120 or above or your diastolic is 80 or above on several occasions, you should discuss this with your family physician.

5. **E = Estimate your cardiac risk.** Several internet-based calculators will estimate your risk of developing heart disease over the next ten years and compare your risk to others of the same age. A heart-risk calculator from the AHA and the American College of Cardiology (ACC) is at tinyurl.com/r9k2q7r. Also, Mayo Clinic has an easy-to-use one at tinyurl.com/vuyx45f.

These ABCDEs will help you determine your risk factors for heart disease. If you have *any* of them, before you even think about a natural medicine, *many* lifestyle interventions are safe and effective at increasing heart health and reducing the risks of cardiovascular disease and premature death. In chapter 3, "What's More Effective Than *Any* Natural Medicine?," and chapter 5, "An Overall Approach to Wellness and Multivitamins," I review these strategies in more depth. Dr. Phil Bishop and I discuss them in detail in our book, *Fit over 50: Make Simple Choices Today for a Healthier, Happier You.*

Here's why it's so critical to know and implement these tactics: 2018 research revealed that five lifestyle choices increase the life expectancy of the average fifty-year-old an average of thirteen years—a whopping 26 percent increase![24] They are:

1. not smoking

2. maintaining a normal BMI (18.5 to 24.9)

3. doing thirty or more minutes per day of physical activity five days a week

4. having no or limited alcohol intake

5. having a high-quality, primarily plant-based, whole-food, nutrient-dense diet

Furthermore, three-fourths of the premature cardiovascular deaths and half of the premature cancer deaths in the US are attributed to *not* doing these same five things.

There is no reliable evidence that natural medicines add any significant benefit to *any* of these five strategies. And the good news is that even if you don't practice all five of these, the more you do and the sooner you do, the better both your quality of life and your quantity of life—and who doesn't want that?

Since natural medicines don't seem to help in the prevention of heart disease, how about those conditions that can lead to heart attack or stroke? Of the three key risk factors for heart disease (high blood pressure/hypertension, high blood cholesterol, and smoking), many supplements are sold to prevent or treat the first two.

Natural Medicines for HBP/HTN

Because there are so many studies and so much misinformation on this topic, let me just cut to the chase and quote the experts at *Natural Medicines*™:

> The role of natural medicines for treating or preventing hypertension is confusing and contradictory. . . . Based on existing evidence, there is no natural medicine that is appropriate as an alternative for patients who need conventional antihypertensive drug therapy. And while many natural medicines have been shown to lower blood pressure in clinical trials, most have not been shown to improve what matters most—cardiovascular outcomes. Nonetheless, certain non-drug approaches including dietary and lifestyle changes, which may include supplements in some cases, are appropriate

for many patients. . . . Dietary interventions have demonstrated the most benefit on blood pressure and might also reduce cardiovascular events and cardiovascular mortality. Such interventions include increased dietary intake of fish, fiber, and potassium, as well as moderate portions of dark chocolate. Adding a natural medicine as adjunctive therapy might be appropriate for some groups of patients. For example, drinking black, green, or hibiscus tea, or consuming pomegranate juice or fermented milk, might provide additive blood pressure reduction. Also, taking fish oil supplements could be beneficial.

DARK CHOCOLATE FLAVONOIDS. The AHA reports, "Every year, Americans spend $22 billion on chocolate."[25] I won't be discussing either milk chocolate or white chocolate, for neither are heart healthy. White chocolate is made with a blend of sugar, cocoa butter, milk products, vanilla, and a fatty substance called lecithin. Technically, white chocolate is not even a chocolate!

Most dark chocolate is high in flavonoids, particularly a subtype called flavanols that is associated with a lower risk of heart disease. *Natural Medicines* explains, "Chocolate is made from cocoa beans, the seeds from the cocoa tree, which is found in tropical climates. The bean powder is a source of the flavanols found in dark unprocessed chocolate, cocoa beverages, and in processed chocolate products in smaller amounts." Although dark chocolate and milk chocolate are both made with cocoa powder and cocoa butter, dark chocolate has a much higher concentration of flavanols because milk chocolate includes milk and typically a larger amount of sugar.

But is dark chocolate heart healthy? ConsumerLab.com points out, "Cocoa-based products are advertised and sold to make you believe that they can provide modest potential benefits regarding blood flow, blood pressure, cholesterol levels, heart health, improved memory and cognition, fewer skin wrinkles, and better blood sugar control." But as you're learning, the advertising is often far from the truth.

The AHA quotes Alice H. Lichtenstein, DSc, of Tufts University in Boston, who sums up the science on the topic: "While dark chocolate has more flavanols than other types of chocolate, the data to suggest there is enough to have a health effect is thin at this point."[26]

Natural Medicines rates cocoa as "Possibly Safe" when used in moderate amounts or in amounts commonly found in foods. As for the various indications, they rate it as "Possibly Effective" for cardiovascular disease and hypertension, "Possibly Ineffective" for hypercholesterolemia, and "Insufficient Evidence" for aging skin, cognitive function, or diabetes.

If you are considering cocoa or dark chocolate for heart health, there are three key issues you need to consider. First and most importantly, as explained by ConsumerLab, "Be careful! Many popular cocoa powders, cacao nibs, and some dark chocolates are contaminated with high levels of cadmium, a toxic heavy metal . . . exceeding established limits for cadmium and representing significant and unnecessary exposure to cadmium. Fortunately, we were able to identify a few great products that minimize cadmium exposure, maximize flavanols, offer superior value, and even minimize calories without sacrificing flavor."

Why the concern?

Cadmium is a probable carcinogen (i.e., cancer-causing agent), can be toxic to the kidneys, can soften the bones, and may affect fetal development. Cadmium accumulates in the body due to its long biological half-life in humans of 10 to 35 years. . . . The cadmium concentrations in many cocoa powders tested by ConsumerLab were 10 to 20 times higher than in cadmium-rich foods [such as peanuts or sunflower seeds]. . . . Unfortunately, the US government has not set a limit for cadmium in supplements or foods. The European Union has established a cadmium limit . . . which most cocoa powders tested in this review would violate.

Second, ConsumerLab advises, "Although cocoa and chocolate products are generally safe, it may be best to limit consumption of products due to contaminants as well as calories. Be aware that the caffeine and theobromine in cocoa products may cause side effects as well as interfere with the actions of certain drugs. Cocoa and chocolate products may also trigger migraines in some people and may trigger allergic contact dermatitis in nickel-sensitive individuals. People with milk allergies should be aware that dark chocolate bars may contain milk."

Third, be aware that the "percent cocoa" or "percent cacao" indicated on a label, as explained by ConsumerLab, "reflects the total amount of cocoa powder plus cocoa butter relative to all other ingredients. As sugar is the only other ingredient in dark chocolate, 'percent cocoa' in dark chocolate tells you the percent that is not sugar. However, as manufacturers typically don't disclose the ratio of cocoa powder to cocoa butter in their chocolates, the 'percent cocoa' is only a rough indicator of how much cocoa powder is in a product and how flavanol-rich the chocolate may be."

These are all reasons to have a third-party testing lab on your side. For example, Labdoor gave very poor ratings to each of the eleven popular dark chocolate products it tested. The best three received a "D-minus" rating:

- *Ghirardelli® Twilight Delight Intense Dark 72% Cacao*
- *Lindt® 70% Cocoa Excellence Dark Chocolate Bar*
- *See's Candies® Premium Dark Chocolate 62% Cacao Bar*

An "F" rating went to the remaining eight products tested:

- *Godiva® 72% Cacao Dark Chocolate Bar*
- *365 Everyday™ Value Organic Dark Chocolate Bar*
- *Trader Joe's® Dark Chocolate Bar*
- *Hershey's® Kisses Special Dark Chocolate Classic*
- *Hershey's® Special Dark Chocolate Bar*
- *Dove® Silky Smooth Dark Chocolate Promises*
- *Cadbury® Royal Dark Indulgent Semi-Sweet*
- *M&M's® Dark Chocolate*[27]

ConsumerLab points out that for cardiovascular health, clinical studies suggest 200 to 900 mg per day of flavanols are needed.

If you are just after flavanols, you'll generally get the most flavanols with the least cadmium contamination and calories from supplements made from cocoa extracts and, among these, the ones with the highest concentration of flavanols is *CocoaVia™ vegetarian capsules* . . . our "Top Pick" among supplements. This product promises 450 mg of flavanols in a daily serving of 2 capsules for $1.33; however, we found an even greater amount of flavanols (600.4 mg) in this same product. This is a reasonable cost for flavanols, with each 200 mg of flavanols costing 59 cents (or just 44 cents based on the amount found).

More recently ConsumerLab wrote:

We tested several powdered *CocoaVia™* products of varying flavors—each listing 450 mg of flavanols per packet. The powder is to be added to drinks, such as milk or coffee, or to foods, like oatmeal or yogurt. All of the products passed our testing and we found the powders to mix easily into liquids. There are two dark chocolate versions (sweetened and unsweetened) and each was found to contain about 1 mcg of cadmium per packet, which is relatively low considering their enormous flavanol content. The original flavor (which is a bit bitter) and cran-raspberry (which is tart and sweet) do not have a chocolate flavor but contain virtually no cadmium (0.01 mcg or less per packet). The dark chocolate versions have a rich dark chocolate taste. The unsweetened version is a bit bitter, but we found it to pack a whopping 753.5 mg of flavanols per packet, which made it our "Top Pick." The sweetened version, which includes sucralose (which is non-caloric), is mildly sweet and was found to provide 497.1 mg of flavanols, which is still quite impressive.

ConsumerLab has a couple of "Top Picks" to consider for dark chocolate products:

If you love strong dark chocolate, don't need it to be sweet, want plenty of flavanols and minimal cadmium contamination, the clear winner, and a "Top Pick" for dark chocolates, is *Montezuma's® Dark Chocolate Absolute Black—100% Cocoa*, which is from England. Compare this with *Trader Joe's® The Dark Chocolate Lover's Chocolate Bar—85% Cacao* (tested in 2017) which had the next highest concentration of flavanols but 12 times as much cadmium . . . the most cadmium in any dark chocolate we tested. . . .

Although *Trader Joe's® Dark Chocolate Lover's Bar* was a cadmium disaster [given an "F" rating by Labdoor] and the two Trader Joe's® cocoa powders in our review were also among the worst in terms of cadmium, this is not the case with *Trader Joe's® Pound Plus—72% Cacao Dark Chocolate*, which is our other "Top Pick" for dark chocolates—for people who like dark chocolate a little sweet. In addition to being the least expensive dark chocolate by far ($4.99 for a huge, 500 gram [1.1 pound] bar), it, like *Montezuma's®*, was among the lowest in cadmium . . . and fairly high in flavanols. Despite containing sugar, it provides fewer calories than many other bars.

ConsumerLab's "Top Pick" among dark chocolate chips is "*Guittard®*
Extra Dark Chocolate Baking Chips—63% Cacao because these chips
provide 81 percent more flavanols per gram than *Ghirardelli® Chocolate*
Premium Baking Chips—60% Cacao (9.6 mg vs. 5.3 mg) and cost a bit
less. However, *Guittard®* does contain a bit more cadmium per gram . . .
making a 15-gram serving exceed the limit in Canada for children, but not
for adults. For children, the *Ghirardelli®* chips may be preferable."

ConsumerLab warns, "A conundrum with cocoa/cacao powders is that
those with the highest flavanol concentrations tend to be the most contaminated with cadmium [and are, consequently, 'Not Approved' by Consu-
merLab]. Conversely, those with little cadmium contamination [and 'Approved' by ConsumerLab] tend to have low flavanol levels. And then there
is the worst of both worlds, a product very low in flavanols but relatively
high in cadmium, as exemplified by *Hershey's® Cocoa Special Dark*. . . .
Fortunately, there is a middle ground, which is where we found our 'Top
Pick': *Ghirardelli® Chocolate Premium Baking Cocoa—100% Cocoa*."

FISH OIL (OMEGA-3 FATTY ACIDS). The most popular of the natural
medicines for heart health is fish oils, which come from a variety of marine
life, including mackerel, herring, tuna, halibut, salmon, and cod liver. Fish
oil is an excellent dietary source of omega-3 fatty acids, also known as n-3
fatty acids. Eicosapentaenoic acid (EPA) and docosahexaenoic acid (DHA)
are two omega-3 fatty acids found in fish oil that have been extensively
studied in humans. In its 2020 "Survey of Supplement Users," Consumer-
Lab reported that fish oil was the second most popular natural medicine,
used by about 56 percent of their respondents.

These numbers may go up based upon extensive publicity in early 2020
surrounding the publication of a study that followed nearly half a million
UK adults (40 to 69 years old) for eight to twelve years. The researchers
reported, "Habitual use of fish oil seems to be associated with a lower risk
of all-cause and CVD mortality and to provide a marginal benefit against
CVD events [heart attacks and strokes] among the general population."[28]

As an observational study, it can only show an association and not
cause and effect. In other words, we can't know for sure if it was the fish
oil supplements alone or something else that had the positive outcomes.
"But," the authors told CNN, "our analysis of the data showed that the

benefits were independent of factors including age, sex, lifestyle habits, diet, medication and other supplement use." Nevertheless, the study did show "the fish oil users were less likely to be current smokers and more likely to engage in physical activity and eat oily fish, which may be a marker of other healthy dietary habits."[29]

Natural Medicines rates fish oil as "Effective" for hypertriglyceridemia; "Possibly Effective" for use after angioplasty, coronary artery bypass surgery, and heart transplant; "Possibly Effective" for heart failure and hypertension; "Insufficient Evidence" for CVD, dyslipidemia, and stroke; and "Possibly Ineffective" for angina, atrial fibrillation, cerebrovascular disease, and peripheral artery disease.

Of course, prior to using fish oil with any of these conditions, you'll want to discuss this with your family physician, cardiologist, or pharmacist.

However, when it comes to heart health in general, AARP® writes, "Even those who regularly pop little more than a multivitamin might be wondering if they should be taking fish oil—what with the constant news about how omega-3 fatty acids might help our health. And at least ten percent of all Americans already take the supplement hoping to keep their hearts strong. But can popping such a pill really protect your ticker?"[30]

Since randomized trials are more likely to shed light on any particular intervention, Deepak Bhatt, MD, executive director of interventional cardiovascular programs at Brigham and Women's Hospital in Boston, told AARP®, "The data to date, if one looks [only] at large randomized clinical trials, which is the highest level of evidence, shows that [fish oil] supplements haven't been found to have any significant cardiovascular benefit."[31]

Natural Medicines agrees, concluding, "Overall, best evidence to date show that fish oil supplements, typically taken in doses of 1 gram daily, are not beneficial for primary or secondary prevention of CVD. Ongoing trials are evaluating whether taking fish oil supplements in higher doses of 3 to 4 grams daily is beneficial. Dietary fish oil might be beneficial for primary or secondary prevention, but benefits are probably modest at best. Still, people should continue to eat fish and other foods that provide omega-3 fatty acids, as these foods make up part of a healthy diet."

JAMA Internal Medicine featured a review done on fish oil research published in major journals over a seven-year period and reported that in twenty-two of the twenty-four studies fish oil showed no benefit.[32] The NCCIH bluntly adds, "Research indicates that omega-3 supplements don't reduce heart disease."[33] AARP® advises, "Doctors agree: If you're healthy and at low risk for heart disease, the best way to get any omega-3s—or any nutrient—is from the food you eat. . . . Time spent in front of a plate of salmon—or another fatty fish brimming with omega-3s—is time not spent stopping at the local fast food drive-thru for a burger and fries. As Matt Budoff, MD, a cardiologist affiliated with UCLA Medical Center, puts it: 'Fish is a smart replacement for bad things.'"[34]

The AHA recommends[35] "two servings of fish a week (3.5 ounces per cooked serving), preferably the fatty kind that's rich in omega-3s. They say that other good sources—besides salmon—include mackerel, herring, lake trout, sardines, and albacore tuna. Vegetarians, people with allergies, or those who dislike seafood can shop for plant-based sources of omega-3 fatty acid, including vegetables (Brussels sprouts and spinach), walnuts, flaxseed, and pumpkin seeds."[36]

But remember, there are some cautions regarding fish. As *Natural Medicines* points out, it is "Possibly Unsafe" when "fish oil from dietary sources is consumed in large amounts. . . . Fatty fish can contain significant amounts of toxins such as mercury, polychlorinated biphenyls (PCBs), dioxin, and dioxin-related compounds. Very frequent consumption of contaminated fish can cause adverse effects."

Furthermore, "Women who are pregnant or who may become pregnant, and nursing mothers should avoid shark, swordfish, king mackerel, and tilefish (also called *golden bass* or *golden snapper*), as these may contain high levels of methylmercury. They should also limit consumption of other fish to 12 ounces/week (about 3 to 4 servings/week)." Because of these warnings, many consumers are choosing fish oil supplements for a wide variety of indications, including heart health. The US omega-3 supplement market size was valued at over $2 billion in 2018.

Some over-the-counter fish oil products have been found to be contaminated, rancid, or suffer from labeling issues. *Natural Medicines* suggests, "Taking fish oil with meals or freezing the capsules seems to help decrease some side effects like GI upset or fish aftertaste especially after burping." Before purchasing a fish oil product, and this is critical, be sure to look at the product reviews of ConsumerLab, Labdoor, or *Natural Medicines* to find products that have been independently quality tested.

In a September 2020 review of fish oil and omega-3 supplements, ConsumerLab "Approved" twenty-six products for quality (out of twenty-eight tested)—meaning that they met labeling requirements and passed quality testing, meeting requirements for freshness and purity (i.e., lack of contamination by heavy metals), containing their claimed amounts of omega-3 fatty acids, and, if enteric coated, disintegrating properly—including products from *GNC*, *Kirkland Signature*™ [Costco®], *Life Extension®*, *Minami Garden of Life®*, *Solgar®*, and *Spring Valley*™ [Walmart]. I discuss ConsumerLab's "Top Picks" for fish oil in chapter 8, "Cholesterol and Dyslipidemia."

Natural Medicines lists 12 USP®-"Verified" products, all of which are NMBER® rated 10 out of 10, including products from *Kirkland Signature*™, *Nature Made®*, *Sunmark®*, and *Berkley and Jensen®*.

Labdoor lists seven "Certified" products and gives a quality rating above a "C" rating (a "B" or "B-minus" rating) to only three products out of fifty-one products tested (sixteen rated "C," twenty-five rated "D," and eight rated "F"). Labdoor reported, "Label accuracy was a major issue for fish oil supplements. Total omega-3 content ranged from -60.0 percent to +62.5 percent versus their stated label claims."

Labdoor added, "Chewable and liquid-formulated fish oil supplements contained much lower EPA + DHA concentration than their softgel counterparts." Even more concerning, "All but four products contained measurable amounts of mercury, with three products recording 50 percent or greater of the allowable mercury content/serving. The majority of products passed oxidation (freshness) assays, although 14 of 54 products recorded peroxide levels (measure of primary oxidation) at or above the upper limit."[37]

GOED (the Global Organization for EPA and DHA, a fish oil trade group) funded its own study of popular US fish oil supplements and found that nearly half of seventeen tested products failed one or more quality tests.[38] Two of the products that passed testing were also "Approved" by ConsumerLab, while none that failed GOED's tests had been "Approved" by ConsumerLab.

Obviously, if you choose to take fish oil, be sure to pick a product that is ConsumerLab "Approved," "USP®-Verified," NMBER rated 9 or 10 out of 10, or Labdoor "Certified" with a rating of "B-minus" or higher.

As to the following chart, it's remarkable to me the myriad natural approaches that have been studied for hypertension—the vast majority of which have not panned out. More detailed information is available from ConsumerLab.com and *Natural Medicines*.

Natural Interventions and Medicines for Hypertension (HTN), Coronary Heart Disease (CHD) or Coronary Artery Disease (CAD), Cardiovascular Disease (CVD), and Congestive Heart Failure (CHF)

Safety / Effective	Likely Safe	Possibly Safe
Effective	★★★★★ • Avoid tobacco products (CAD,CVD,CHD,HTN) • Lifestyle changes (CAD,CVD,CHD,HTN) • Maintain a normal BMI (CAD,CVD,CHD,HTN) • Nutrient-dense foods (fruits, vegetables, lean protein, heart-healthy fats) (CAD,CVD,CHD,HTN) • Regular exercise (CAD,CVD,CHD,HTN) • Restful sleep (CAD,CVD,CHD,HTN)	★★
Likely Effective	★★★★ • Black psyllium (CHD) • DASH diet (HTN) • Oats (CVD) • Potassium (HTN) • Reduce stress (CAD,CVD,CHD,HTN)	★★
Possibly Effective	★★ • Alpha-linolenic acid (CVD,HTN) • Anti-inflammatory diet (CVD) • Blond psyllium (HTN) • Calcium (from foods) (HTN) • Canola oil (CHD) • Cocoa (CVD,HTN) • Coenzyme Q10 (CHF)	★ • Alcohol (beer/wine) in moderation (CHF,CVD,HTN) • Black seed (HTN) • Blue-green algae (HTN) • Chitosan (HTN) • Conjugated linoleic acid (CLA) (HTN)

Possibly Effective	• DASH diet (CVD) • Docosahexaenoic Acid (DHA) (CHD) • Eicosapentaenoic Acid (EPA) (CHD,CVD) • Fish oil (CHF,HTN) • Flaxseed (ground) (HTN) • Folic acid (vitamin B9) (HTN) • Gamma-aminobutyric acid (GABA) (HTN) • Garlic (HTN) • Green tea (CHD,HTN) • Guar gum (HTN) • Iron (CHF) • L-Carnitine (CHF) • Magnesium (CHD) • Meditation (HTN) • Mediterranean diet (CVD) • Music therapy (HTN) • Olive (CVD,HTN) • Propionyl-L-carnitine (CHD,CHF,CVD) • Relaxation therapy (HTN) • Ribose (CAD,CHF,CVD) • Sunflower oil (CHD,CVD) • Tai chi (CHF,HTN) • Vegetarian diet (HTN) • Vitamin D (CHF) • Vitamins, prenatal (CHD) • Yoga (HTN)	• Fermented Milk (HTN) • Hawthorn (CHF) • Hibiscus (HTN) • L-arginine (HTN) • L-Citrulline (CHF) • Lycopene (HTN) • Melatonin (HTN) • Pomegranate (HTN) • Red yeast rice (CVD) • Sesame (HTN) • Soy (HTN) • Sweet orange (HTN) • Taurine (CHF) • Vitamin C (HTN) • Wheat bran (HTN)

Insufficient evidence for safety or effectiveness AND/OR evidence for lack of safety or effectiveness

 • Acetyl-L-carnitine (HTN) • Aconite (CHF) • Acupuncture (HTN) • Alpha-lipoic acid (CHF,HTN) • American ginseng (HTN) • Artichoke (HTN) • Asparagus (HTN) • Astragalus (CHF) • Basil (HTN) • Beet (HTN) • Berberine (CHD,CHF) • Beta-carotene (CVD) • Beta-glucans (HTN) • Bilberry (HTN)	• Biofeedback (HTN) • Black cohosh (CVD) • Black currant (HTN) • Black tea (CHD,HTN) • Blueberry (HTN) • Calcium (CHF,CVD,HTN) • Canola oil (HTN) • Cardamom (HTN) • Carnosine (CHF) • Casein peptides (HTN) • Casein protein (HTN) • Celery seed (HTN) • Chanca piedra (HTN) • Chia (HTN) • Chiropractic (HTN)

- Chlorella (HTN)
- Chokeberry (CAD,CHD)
- Choline (CVD)
- Cocoa (CHF)
- Coconut oil (CHD)
- Coconut water (HTN)
- Cod liver oil (HTN)
- Coenzyme Q10 (CVD,HTN)
- Coffee (HTN)
- Coleus (HTN)
- Cranberry (CAD)
- Creatine (CHF)
- Cupping (HTN)
- Danshen (CHD,CVD,HTN)
- DHEA (CVD)
- Docosahexaenoic acid (DHA) (HTN)
- Dong quai (CHD)
- EDTA (CAD)
- Eicosapentaenoic acid (EPA) (HTN)
- Elderberry fruit extract (CVD)
- Elderberry leaves or stems (CVD)
- Eleuthero (Siberian ginseng) (CHD)
- English walnut (CHD)
- Equol (CVD)
- Fish oil (CVD)
- Flaxseed (ground) (CVD)
- Flaxseed oil (CVD,HTN)
- Folic acid (vitamin B9) (CHD)
- Folic acid (vitamin B9) (CVD)
- Foxglove (CHF)
- Gamma linolenic acid (GLA) (HTN)
- Garlic (CHD)
- Ginger (HTN)
- Ginkgo (CVD,HTN)
- Glucomannan (HTN)
- Glucosamine HCL (CVD)
- Glucosamine sulfate (CVD)
- Grape (CVD,HTN)
- Green tea (CVD)
- Guava (HTN)
- Hawthorn (HTN)
- Hesperidin (HTN)
- Hydrotherapy (CHF)
- Hydroxymethylbutyrate (HMB) (HTN)
- Hypnotherapy (HTN)
- Indian snakeroot (HTN)
- Iridology (for diagnosis)
- Java tea (HTN)
- Ketogenic diet (HTN)
- Kiwi (HTN)
- Kudzu (CHD,CHF,HTN)
- L-Arginine (CHD,CHF)
- Lavender (HTN)
- L-Carnitine (CHD)
- L-Citrulline (HTN)
- Lemon (HTN)
- Lutein (CVD)
- Lycopene (CVD,HTN)
- Magnesium (CVD,HTN)
- Maritime pine (CAD,CHF,HTN)
- Massage (HTN)
- Meditation (CHF,CVD)
- Mediterranean diet (HTN)
- Motherwort (HTN)
- Moxibustion (HTN)
- Multivitamins (CVD,HTN)
- Music therapy (CVD)
- N-acetyl glucosamine (NAG) (CVD)
- Niacin (vitamin B3) (CVD)
- Nicotinamide riboside (HTN)
- Omega-6 fatty acids (CVD)
- Oolong tea (HTN)
- Organic food (CVD,HTN)
- Ornish diet (CVD,HTN)
- Paleo diet (HTN)
- Panax ginseng (CHF,HTN)
- Passionflower (CHF)
- Pea protein (HTN)
- Physical therapy (CHF)
- Policosanol (CHD)
- Prayer and healing, distant (CVD,HTN)
- Pomegranate (CHD)
- Progesterone (CVD)
- Qi gong (CAD)
- Quercetin (CVD,HTN)
- Red yeast rice (HTN)
- Reishi mushroom extract (CHD,HTN)
- Reishi mushroom powder (CHD,HTN)
- Relaxation therapy (CHF)
- Reservatrol (CVD)
- Riboflavin (vitamin B2) (HTN)
- Saccharomyces boulardii (CHF)

• Safflower flower (HTN)	• Terminalia (CHD,CHF)
• Safflower seed oil (HTN)	• Tomato extract (CVD,HTN)
• Saffron (HTN)	• Tyrosine (HTN)
• Sea buckthorn (CVD,HTN)	• Vegetarian diet (CVD)
• Selenium (CHF,CVD)	• Vitamin B3 (niacin) (CVD)
• Shirodhara (HTN)	• Vitamin B6 (pyridoxine)
• Sour cherry (HTN)	(CVD,HTN)
• Soy (CVD)	• Vitamin C (CVD)
• Squill (CHD)	• Vitamin D (CVD,HTN)
• Star of Bethlehem (CHF)	• Vitamin K (CHD)
• Stem cell therapy (direct to consumer for CHF)	• Vitamin E (CHF,CVD,HTN)
• Stevia (HTN)	• Whey protein (HTN)
• Sunflower oil (HTN)	• Yoga (CHF,CVD)
• Sweet almond (CHD)	• Yogurt (CVD)
• Tai chi (CHD)	• Yucca (HTN)
• Taurine (HTN)	• Zinc (CHD)

Most of the recommendations in the chart are based on the "Safety and Effectiveness Ratings" contained in *Natural Medicines™* and explained in chapter 4 of this book. They assume the use of high-quality, uncontaminated products and the use of typical doses. Keep in mind that some products are never appropriate for some patients due to concomitant disease states, potential drug interactions, or other clinical factors. Details are available at *Natural Medicines™*.

15

Immune Health

O ver the years, countless dietary supplements, alternative remedies, and foods have been touted as immune-system boosters," begins a review on "Boosting Your Immune System" in *Consumer Reports*. "In fact, more than 1,000 supplements currently on the US market are claimed to have a positive effect on immunity."[1] The advertising must be working, as the fourth most common reason that people in the age groups eighteen to thirty-four and thirty-five to fifty-four take natural medicines is for "immune health," "immune support," or to boost "immune response." Twenty-five percent and 31 percent respectively in each age group take these supplements daily.[2] This represented almost forty million Americans in 2018.[3] Unfortunately, many of them may be wasting hard-earned dollars. I'll explain why, but first, let's review some basics.

Each of us must contend with a never-ending onslaught of potentially dangerous microorganisms (germs). The system that guards our bodies utilizes a wide variety of defenses that are collectively called the *immune system*. Likely you've heard of diseases that result in immune deficiency—the best known of which is acquired immune deficiency syndrome (AIDS), which is caused by the human immunodeficiency virus (HIV). People with immune deficiency are susceptible to many different infectious microorganisms that most healthy persons can fight off.

Can You Boost Your Immune System?

Of course, healthy people get sick from time to time when infections manage to slip by or through our defenses—while others find themselves frequently coming down with illnesses like colds. Often people in these categories want to find treatments that can strengthen their immune system. Unfortunately, this is much easier said than done.

The *Natural and Alternative Treatments™ Encyclopedia* explains,

> Many natural products are said to boost general immunity. However, while we can scientifically study the effect of a single treatment on a single illness, at the present state of knowledge, there is no way we can even know that a treatment strengthens the immune system in general. Scientists can measure the effects of an herb on individual white blood cell types and note changes in activity, but they do not know how to interpret the results of those measurements as a whole. After all, the immune system is a system, and systems are notoriously complicated to analyze. Current knowledge does not allow us to predict the ultimate effect of fine changes in the parts.[4]

"The idea of boosting your immunity is enticing, but the ability to do so has proved elusive for several reasons," writes *Harvard Health*. "The immune system is precisely that—a system, not a single entity. To function well, it requires balance and harmony. There is still much that researchers don't know about the intricacies and interconnectedness of the immune response. For now, there are no scientifically proven direct links [to] enhanced immune function." They add, "Many products on store shelves claim to boost or support immunity. But the concept of boosting immunity actually makes little sense scientifically."[5]

Because consumers are becoming more aware that supplements have not been shown to boost the immune system, supplement makers are increasingly using terms such as "fine-tuning the immune system" or "supporting immune health" or "supplementing immune modulators." The *Natural and Alternative Treatments™ Encyclopedia* opines, "Does such a treatment exist? No one really knows, although claims abound."[6]

Harriet H. Hall, MD, an editor and weekly contributor to the blog at Science-Based Medicine and a contributor to QuackWatch is more explicit: "Do our immune systems need help? Walk into any health foods store. Browse the Internet. You will find a multitude of diet supplements advertised to 'boost your immune system,' or 'support immune function.' Do they work? Will they keep you healthier or reduce your chances of catching infectious diseases? . . . Their claims are not supported by science. For normal people whose nutrition is adequate, no high-quality clinical study has ever shown that any intervention led to any meaningful improvement in immune function or to any decrease in the rate of disease."[7]

A review article in *EveryDay Health* was titled more emphatically: "Immune System Boosters—One of the Biggest Scams Around." The report was authored by Ed Zimney, MD, a former FDA medical officer and branch chief, regulating prescription drug advertising at a national level, who wrote, "There are no effective immune system booster products. I know that the Internet is awash in products claiming to enhance the immune system, but there's simply no scientific evidence that they work. . . . All the millions that people spend on these products does nothing more than fill the coffers of the unscrupulous companies peddling them (how these people even sleep at night is beyond me!)."[8]

Marvin M. Lipman, MD, the chief medical adviser to Consumer Reports, says, "The proof of any purported immune booster is whether it can increase your resistance to infections. . . . No dietary supplement or alternative remedy has so far been shown to do so."[9] David Nieman, DrPH, a researcher in immunology and director of the Human Performance Laboratory at Appalachian State University, says, "You can't boost [the immune system] by adding nutrients." He adds, "Most immune system claims are 'misleading.' You can't strengthen the immune system by adding extra vitamins or minerals unless the person has a severe deficiency as a result of a disease like HIV."[10]

I mentioned HIV/AIDS, one of the most well-known and dangerous immune deficiency diseases. Dr. Zimney points out, "The people who do have HIV/AIDS can attest to just how hard it is to enhance their immune systems (in fact, the only way is by eliminating the virus with antiviral therapy). If any of these so-called immune system boosters really worked, they'd immediately be used in the treatment of HIV/AIDS (but they don't and therefore aren't)."[11]

False Advertising Yet Again

As consumers, we are bombarded by dubious health information—especially on the internet. In 2019, Brazilian researchers evaluated the top 185 web pages from a Google search on "boost immunity" in terms of the specific "boosters" mentioned and reported. "Of the 37 approaches to boost immunity recorded, the top ones were:

- diet (77 percent of web pages),
- fruit (69 percent),
- vitamins (67 percent),
- antioxidants (52 percent),
- probiotics (51 percent),
- minerals (50 percent), and
- vitamin C (49 percent)."[12]

They then evaluated the websites and found commercial websites had a significant "over-representation of 'minerals' and 'supplements,'" and "the information quality of commercial websites, as assessed by two tools that assess webpages' transparency and trustworthiness is low."[13]

Another study reported that among health websites, retail websites presenting information on products they were selling had the lowest level of medical accuracy (only 9 percent).[14]

So, buyer beware! Even with the limited scope of regulations on natural medicines, if there are, in fact, no studies showing they work to significantly reduce the risk of disease or illness, then you'd be right to expect plenty of false advertising. And you'd be correct. According to Dr. Hall, "The FDA and the FTC have been cracking down on dubious 'immune boosting' product claims. For instance, Andrew Weil's website was recently ordered to stop claiming that its products could help prevent swine flu and colds."[15] Following are just a few other actions the federal government took against the more egregious false claims:

- CVS/Pharmacy™ paid nearly $2.8 million in consumer refunds to settle Federal Trade Commission (FTC) charges of unsubstantiated advertising of *AirShield*® "Immune Boosting" Supplement. The

FTC order "barred CVS from making claims that any CVS-brand food, drug, or dietary supplement can reduce the risk of or prevent colds, protect against cold viruses in crowded places, fight germs, or boost the immune system unless the claims are true and backed by scientific evidence."[16]

- Florida-based supplement sellers NextGen Nutritionals, Strictly Health, and Cyber Business Technology settled FTC false advertising charges—including a judgment of over $1.3 million for making "immune support and disease prevention . . . claims" for several supplements—claims that were "false or unsubstantiated." One product was publicized to be able to "super-charge your immune system" and "defeat the common cold, flu, viruses and deadly diseases." The fabricated advertisements cited "rock-solid science" and claimed one supplement "works wonders" against cold, flu, and viruses and "reduces health-related time-off from work by a whopping 97 percent."[17]

- *Emergen-C®* settled a false advertising lawsuit. Alacer Corporation, its marketers, agreed "to pay $6.45 million to settle a class action lawsuit which charged the company made false claims that the vitamin C supplement could boost immunity." ConsumerLab.com reported, "Statements made in advertisements and on *Emergen-C®* packaging [claimed] that the supplement could 'power up' the immune system. . . . While the company maintains it made no false claims, it will offer payments to anyone who purchased various *Emergen-C®* products."

- ConsumerLab also reported, "The maker of the popular *Airborne® Effervescent Health Formula*, an effervescent tablet marketed as a cold prevention and treatment remedy, has agreed to pay up to $30 million to settle FTC charges that it did not have adequate evidence to support its advertising claims." According to the FTC's complaint, "There is no competent and reliable scientific evidence to support the claims made by the defendants that *Airborne®* tablets can prevent or reduce the risk of colds, sickness, or infection; protect against or help fight germs; reduce the severity or duration of a cold; and protect against colds, sickness, or infection in crowded places such as airplanes, offices, or schools."

- "Dannon® Company settled a class-action lawsuit alleging that company engaged in false advertising by touting the health benefits of yogurt products," reported the *Chicago Tribune*. "Dannon®, which denied wrongdoing, agreed to set up a $35 million fund for reimbursing consumers. Labels that once claimed, 'A positive effect on your digestive tract's immune system' instead are to say the yogurt will 'interact' with that system."[18]

As a result of these actions, advertisers and supplement makers are changing their tactics and increasingly saying there is plenty of evidence in animals and humans that their product has been shown to "boost immune response." They are correct that there is indeed some supporting research. Still, it almost exclusively measures this or that blood level of immune components (like infection-fighting immunoglobulin or white blood cells). This research does not show improvement of the immune system as a whole, and even more importantly, has not shown any positive clinical outcomes such as fewer cases of influenza or colds.

Family physician David Rakel, MD, director of integrative medicine at the University of Wisconsin at Madison, explains this concept further: "Herbs and nutrients can help increase the numbers of chemicals and cells in the immune system, but it doesn't always translate to improved immune function." Harvard Medical School adds, "Although some preparations have been found to alter some components of immune function, thus far, there is no evidence that they actually bolster immunity to the point where you are better protected against infection and disease."[19]

Don't Boost—Balance!

What, if anything, has been proven to boost your immunity and prevent disease and death? In 2019, Brazilian researchers looked at a vast amount of data and concluded, "The only evidence-based approach to [boost immunity] is vaccination . . . demonstrated by the enormous success of vaccination in eradicating disease."[20] Dr. Lipman, speaking about immune boosters that increase your resistance to infections, says vaccines can help, but "no dietary supplement or alternative remedy has so far been shown to do so."[21]

Mark Crislip, MD, an infectious disease specialist and chief of infectious diseases at Legacy Health Hospital System in Portland, Oregon, and host of the *QuackCast* podcast, has a great illustration:[22]

> Take the immune system. Please. It is not a bicep that can be made stronger with a little exercise. It is a complex network of cells and proteins. There is no validity to the concept, the myth, of boosting your immune system. Metaphor time: Think of the body as a . . . machine, like a car. . . . You can be properly tuned and maintained, the fluids and gas topped off, the air in the tires at the proper pressure. It will run optimally. You can't over tune the car or fill the tank past capacity. There is an optimum you can't go beyond.

Using the motor analogy, if your oil level gets too low, your engine may not run well or may break. You can fill up the oil to the proper amount, which promotes engine efficiency and life, but extra oil does no good whatsoever, is an unneeded expense, and may do harm. We see this with vitamin D in relation to COVID-19. ConsumerLab writes, "Preliminary studies suggest that people with lower levels of vitamin D are more likely to test positive for the coronavirus, have more severe symptoms (including increased need for intensive care and ventilation), and may have a greater risk of death from COVID-19. Correcting vitamin D may reduce the need for intensive care." But for those with adequate levels of vitamin D, taking extra has no benefit at all in the prevention or treatment of the disease.

According to Glasgow University researchers, "Instead of concentrating on 'boosting' the immune system, a more useful approach might be to think about 'balance,' as a healthy immune system is one that sits in balance." They encourage us to think about our immune systems "as a scale running from 'underactive' to 'overactive.'"[23] As discussed earlier, an underactive immune system is a bad thing. But an overactive immune system may be even worse—as it can start targeting our cells. As a physician, I see this all the time in what are called *autoimmune diseases* such as rheumatoid arthritis and multiple sclerosis.

Dr. Zimney writes, "Let's look at illnesses caused by immune system over-activity. The list here is, unfortunately, huge. How many people do you know who suffer from allergies or asthma? For these people, things in the environment that most people abide without incident cause their immune system to overreact, leaving them suffering miserably." He adds:

> Then we have all the inflammatory diseases: inflammatory bowel disease (Crohn's and ulcerative colitis) . . . and inflammatory skin disease (psoriasis for one). By definition, inflammatory diseases are caused by an overactive immune system. Sometimes these are known as *autoimmune disorders* because the immune system, instead of reacting to foreign material, is reacting to the body's tissues. The list of autoimmune diseases is already quite long, and, every day, new research is showing that more and more illnesses are immune-mediated. . . . . If anything, you'd probably want your immune system dampened down. That's because the treatment for the problems noted above is to try to ratchet down the overactive immune system."[24]

More recent examples of the harm of overactive immune systems include the devastating and very dangerous zoonotic (because they spread from animals to humans) and novel coronavirus epidemics. Severe acute respiratory syndrome coronavirus (SARS-CoV) occurred in 2002. The Middle East respiratory syndrome coronavirus (MERS-CoV) appeared in 2012. COVID-19 (now called SARS-CoV-2) exploded across the globe after starting in China in 2019. In each case, researchers quickly learned the severity of the disease was "associated with an immune response out of control" or "an overreaction of the immune system called a *cytokine storm*." This resulted in "severe pulmonary tissue damage, functional impairment, and reduced lung capacity." Of course, countless deaths occurred—all from immune systems running on overdrive.[25]

The Best Way to Balance Your Immune System

Besides vaccinations, what else can you do that is most effective at supporting, improving, or balancing your immune system? *Harvard Health* observes, "Researchers are exploring the effects of diet, exercise, age, psychological stress, and other factors on the immune response, both in animals and in humans. In the meantime, general healthy-living strategies are a good way to start giving your immune system the upper hand."[26]

The researchers add, "Your first line of defense is to choose a healthy lifestyle. Following general good-health guidelines is the single best step you can take toward naturally keeping your immune system strong and healthy. (I discuss this in more depth in chapter 5, "An Overall Approach to Wellness and Multivitamins.")

Every part of your body, including your immune system, functions better when protected from environmental assaults and bolstered by healthy-living strategies such as these:

- Don't smoke.
- Eat a diet high in fruits and vegetables.
- Exercise regularly.
- Maintain a healthy weight.
- If you drink alcohol, drink only in moderation.
- Get adequate sleep.
- Take steps to avoid infection, such as washing your hands frequently and cooking meats thoroughly.
- Try to minimize stress."[27]

To these, *Consumer Reports* adds:

- Cultivate life's "wow" moments.
- Indulge in a massage.
- Nurture friendships.
- Ease stress.
- Visit a park.[28]

Renee Scola, MD, a primary care physician at Northwestern Memorial Hospital in Chicago, advises, "It's really impossible to boost your immune system instantly by taking a pill. What keeps it healthy are the common-sense things you do on a daily basis: Eating a well-balanced diet, sleeping, exercising, and de-stressing yourself."[29]

Dr. Crislip adds, "With the immune system . . . there are certainly habits that will have everything running suboptimally, and by altering those habits you will get the function close to its theoretical optimum. That is the things you learned in second grade: good diet, exercise, avoid tobacco, a good night's sleep. All the things we know we should do but, the flesh being weak or the Internet being interesting, we often avoid."[30]

Even though I do not have the space to discuss many other natural medicines advertised for immune health, I've included the ratings for some of the more common ones in the following chart. More detailed information is available from ConsumerLab.com and *Natural Medicines*.

Natural Interventions for Immune Health

Safe / Effective	Likely Safe	Possibly Safe
Effective	★★★★★ • Avoid tobacco products • Eat a diet high in fruits and vegetables • Lifestyle changes • Nutrient-dense foods (fruits, vegetables, lean protein, heart-healthy fats) • Regular exercise • Restful sleep • Routine vaccinations • Take steps to avoid infection (e.g., wash hands frequently, cook meats thoroughly)	★★★
Likely Effective	★★★★ • Avoid social isolation • Maintain a normal BMI • Mental stimulation • Nurture friendships • Reduce stress • Spend time outdoors	★★
Possibly Effective	★★★ • Cultivate life's "wow" moments • Massage	★ • Alcohol (beer/wine) in moderation
Insufficient evidence for safety or effectiveness AND/OR evidence for lack of safety or effectiveness		
☹ • Andrographis • Astragalus (Sambucus) • Black tea		• CBD • DHA • Echinacea • Elderberry

• EPA	• Mineral supplements
• Fish oil	• Multivitamins
• Garlic	• N-acetyl cysteine
• Ginger	• Olive oil
• Goldenseal	• Probiotics
• Green tea	• THC (tetrahydrocannabinol)
• Homeopathy	• Turmeric
• Immune "modulators"	• Umckaloabo
• Immune support products	• Vitamin C
• Kombucha	• Zinc
• Marijuana	

Most of the recommendations in the chart are based on the "Safety and Effectiveness Ratings" contained in *Natural Medicines™* and explained in chapter 4 of this book. They assume the use of high-quality, uncontaminated products and the use of typical doses. Keep in mind that some products are never appropriate for some patients due to concomitant disease states, potential drug interactions, or other clinical factors. Details are available at *Natural Medicines™*.

16

Keeping Skin and Nails Young

A 2018 national survey reported the reasons that people are taking natural medicines. The third most popular reason for those eighteen to thirty-four and the fourth most popular reason for those thirty-five to fifty-four was for hair, skin, and/or nails. A striking 28 percent of the former age group and 23 percent of the latter group reported using one or more of these types of products daily.[1] *Consumer Reports* states, "There's no shortage of products on the market that are claimed to thicken hair, remove wrinkles, and fix dry, brittle nails. Among these are a slew of dietary supplements, some topping $100."[2]

Natural medicines for hair, skin, and nail health commonly contain vitamins A, C, or E, coenzyme Q10, or biotin (vitamin B7). For hair, products including manganese and selenium along with fatty acids such as fish oil and flaxseed oil are not uncommon. The companies that are selling these products often advertise that deficiency of these and other nutrients causes unsightly hair, skin, and nail changes that they claim can be prevented or mitigated by their products. What they don't mention is that a deficiency in *any* of these vitamins or minerals is extremely uncommon in the US.

Most dermatologists tell me there's no compelling evidence that natural medicines can make any difference whatsoever for the vast majority of people who have no deficiency in any of these vitamins or supplements. Pieter Cohen, MD, an assistant professor of medicine at Harvard Medical

191

School and an expert on dietary supplements, told *Consumer Reports*, "I'm not aware of any robust data suggesting that any supplements can treat natural, aging-related hair loss or nail damage, or give you healthier skin."[3] Furthermore, there are myriad medical reasons for hair, nail, or skin problems.

As I advise in chapter 13, "Healthy Hair and Hair Loss," if you're experiencing chronic hair, nail, or skin problems for no apparent reason, talk with your family physician or a dermatologist before trying *any* natural medicines. Why? Once again, early treatment is far more effective!

Multivitamins for Skin and Nails

For the reasons I discussed earlier (see chapter 5, "An Overall Approach to Wellness and Multivitamins"), I consider multivitamins to be "Possibly Unsafe" and "Possibly Ineffective" for most consumers. Nevertheless, for those choosing a multivitamin for hair, skin, or nail health, Labdoor tested "Hair Vitamins" and "Certified" *Do Vitamins*® *VitaBeard*®. They gave a "B-plus" rating to *Vitafusion*™ *Gorgeous Hair, Skin, & Nails Multivitamin* and a "B" rating to *Nature's Bounty*® *Optimal Solutions Hair, Skin & Nails*.[4]

One popular product, *SugarBearHair*® *Hair Vitamin*, was not "Approved" by ConsumerLab.com in a 2020 review as the product "contained 160.5 percent of its listed amount of pantothenic acid and 163 percent of its listed amount of vitamin B-6 [pyridoxine]." ConsumerLab advises, "This indicates a high overage of those vitamins but does not pose a health risk. Like other hair and nail formulas, the focus of this product is on its very high dose of biotin (5,000 mcg)." And it is "very expensive," costing "50 cents per gummy." In addition, taking biotin can affect several common lab tests. Read more about biotin later in this chapter.

USP® has "Verified" two multivitamins sold for "hair, skin, and nails" (both are from *Nature Made*® and contain 2,500 mcg of biotin and 100 mg of Vitamin C: *Nature Made*® *Hair, Skin and Nails Gummies* and *Nature Made*® *Hair, Skin and Nails Mini Softgels*).[5] *Natural Medicines*™ lists several "Hair, Skin & Nails Gummies" products that are NMBER® rated 8 out of 10, including products from *Nature's Bounty*®, *Optimal Solutions*, and *Vitamin World*®.

For those who wisely, in my opinion, do not take a multivitamin for hair, skin, or nails, what natural medicine options are there?

Aging Skin and Wrinkles

People spend a lot of money on skincare. On the low side, Statista (a German online portal for statistics) said that in 2019, 1.66 million Americans paid $2,000 or more on skincare products. One-third (33 percent) spent $400 or more, while a whopping 75 percent spent $200 or more.[6] A SkinStore survey reported that the average American woman spent an average of $5 a day toward skincare products (and this does *not* include makeup)—amounting to just under $2,000 a year in 2018. Over a lifetime, SkinStore says, this turns out to be over $200,000 or about ten percent of the average woman's lifetime income. *DermLetter* adds, "It's clear that women are willing to back up their skin with their wallet."[7]

Before we discuss natural medicines for preventing or treating aging skin and wrinkles, I've adapted these commonsense tips from Mayo Clinic for protecting your skin and minimizing premature skin aging or the appearance of wrinkles:[8]

- *Protect your skin from the sun.* Use sunscreen year-round when outdoors.
- *Choose skin-care products with a built-in sun protection factor (SPF) of at least 15.* The American Academy of Dermatology (AAD) recommends using a broad-spectrum sunscreen with an SPF of 30 or more. When selecting UV blocking products, choose those with a broad-spectrum sunscreen—meaning they block both UVA and UVB rays. Always apply generously.
- *Moisturize.* Dry skin shrivels plump skin cells, which can lead to premature fine lines and wrinkles. Moisturizing traps water in your skin, which helps mask tiny lines and creases. It may take a few weeks of regular use of the product before you notice any improvement in your skin. Dr. Griffith shares, "Practically, patients who apply moisturizers over slightly damp extremities after bathing find it easier to form the habit. Most moisturizers marketed for the

face also contain sunscreens, which definitely slows the changes of photoaging."

- *Don't smoke.* Even if you've smoked for years or smoke heavily, you can still improve your skin tone and texture and prevent wrinkles by quitting smoking.
- *Eat a healthy diet.* There is some evidence that certain vitamins in your diet (in foods and *not* in supplements) help protect your skin. More study is needed on the role of nutrition, but it's good to eat plenty of fruits and vegetables.

What about Sunscreens?

One recent concern about sunscreens is the research suggesting that some of the chemicals in sunscreens absorb into your bloodstream after "maximal use." There's no indication so far of any clinical problems with this. As AAD points out, "Just because an ingredient is absorbed into the bloodstream does not mean that it is harmful or unsafe. Most importantly, the study authors and the FDA conclude that consumers should continue to use sunscreen to protect themselves from the sun."

AAD recommends "that everyone seek shade, wear protective clothing—including a lightweight and long-sleeved shirt, pants, a wide-brimmed hat, and sunglasses—and apply a broad-spectrum sunscreen to all exposed skin. These recommendations are based on current scientific evidence—which shows a sunscreen is an effective way to reduce skin cancer risk."[9]

AAD adds, "In addition to chemical sunscreens, people can use physical sunscreens, also known as mineral sunscreens, which act like a shield. They sit on the surface of the skin, primarily deflecting the sun's rays. They include the active ingredients titanium dioxide or zinc oxide and are also recommended for people with sensitive skin."[10] The medical experts at *Up-To-Date* advise, "Pending further data, we continue to advise that patients use sunscreen along with other sun-protection measures."[11]

The Skin Cancer Foundation writes, "Wrinkles, fine lines and pigmentation are inevitable skin woes that often appear as we age. While we like to place blame on getting another year older, the main culprit is photoaging—damage to the skin caused by exposure to sunlight and ultraviolet (UV) light. Responsible for 90 percent of visible changes to the skin, photoaging is a direct result of cumulative sun damage you've been exposed to throughout your life."[12] And, "Photoaging from sunlight also can result in reduced skin elasticity, the degradation of skin texture, and many other signs of skin aging. This has been shown repeatedly, in different parts of the world, over many years, and in many different clinical studies."[13]

Natural Medicines says, "Skin that gets more sun exposure shows far more signs of aging than the less exposed skin. Compare the skin on the outside of the arm with the skin on the underside. Which side looks younger?" They add, "Excessive sun exposure can also lead to more serious conditions including premalignant lesions such as actinic keratoses and malignant lesions such as squamous cell carcinoma, basal cell carcinoma, and malignant melanoma." Also, "The best offense against aging skin is a good defense against sun damage," and "sunscreen is the most effective skin defense on the market."

The use of a broad-spectrum sunscreen dramatically reduces skin damage and aging. Even more importantly, these sunscreens can help prevent melanoma and other types of skin cancer. I usually recommend to ALL of my patients that they apply a sunscreen with an SPF of at least 20 no less than twenty minutes before sun exposure (I call it *Dr. Walt's 20-20 rule*). If you're going to be in the sun, reapply it every two hours after that. Also, protective clothing and a wide-brimmed hat of at least four inches can help. Try to avoid the sun when the rays are most intense, usually between 10:00 a.m. and 4:00 p.m. The bottom line is that you can best prevent premature aging of your skin by staying out of the sun when you can and by using sunscreen when you can't.

Dr. Griffith adds, "The most common query I get in the office is, 'What is the best sunscreen?' My answer: 'The one you will put on. The best sunscreen in the world is not useful if it stays inside the bottle,'" adding, "I recommend a broad-spectrum, water-resistant brand of SPF 30 or higher. In the south, the beach, sweat, and sun are routinely mixed, so water resistance is important. Also, UV protective clothing is easiest for the trunk, especially when swimming."

Most experts now say that concern about vitamin D levels is *not* a good reason to avoid wearing sunscreen. *Natural Medicines* counsels, "While sunscreens do limit the amount of vitamin D produced by the body, the reduction is rarely enough to cause vitamin D deficiency."

Tanning Booths

Avoid tanning booths at all costs. According to the American Society for Dermatologic Surgery (ASDS), "Exposure to the ultraviolet light from tanning beds can impact the skin in a variety of ways—including wrinkles, sunspots or freckles. And for one in every five Americans, this exposure can lead to skin cancer. The use of tanning beds and sun lamps is hazardous because the UV radiation they deliver can damage your skin. Dermatologists highly recommend not using tanning beds and sun lamps. There is growing evidence they may increase your risk of developing melanoma."[14]

AAD points out that tanning beds

- are not safer than the sun,
- make your skin age more quickly,
- can cause eye injuries,
- cannot prevent sunburn, and
- can make stretch marks more visible.

The AAD adds this disturbing information: "Growing evidence indicates that tanning can be addictive. About 20 percent of 18- to 30-year-old white women who use indoor tanning show signs of addiction. They find it hard to stop tanning. When they don't get a steady dose of UV rays, they feel fidgety or depressed."[15]

Natural Medicines for Aging Skin and Wrinkles

Collagen, mainly type I collagen, is a major structural protein of the skin that declines during aging. This leads to your skin thinning and becoming fragile, which increases wrinkling, the risk of bruising, and wound healing disorders. Several topical treatments may restore collagen production in the skin and could hold promise to improve skin health. As a result, as *Natural Medicines* writes, "Aging Baby Boomers have created a *huge* market for skincare products that they hope will 'turn back time.'"

Natural Medicines adds, "There continues to be growth in anti-aging products on the market to address these needs. These products are often called *cosmeceuticals*. They're promoted as being more powerful than regular cosmetics, but not so powerful that they're regulated like drugs. Many come in the form of facial creams or lotions, beefed up with antioxidants and other interesting and sometimes questionable ingredients. Some cosmeceuticals are even taken by mouth. Although many cosmeceuticals are marketed using claims that may sound medical in nature, they are typically regulated as cosmetics or dietary supplements rather than as prescription or over-the-counter drugs."

Natural Medicines points out that "cosmeceuticals . . . do not have the same pre-market approval process as drugs. There are no rigorous safety or effectiveness standards required in order to market a cosmeceutical. Therefore, cosmeceuticals often enter the market without testing or evidence to support safety or to support the claims that are made." Nevertheless, there are some worthy of your consideration.

Topical Retinoids, Adapalene, and Retinols

Currently, prescription products approved for treating aged skin include tretinoin (*Renova*®, *Retin-A*®) and tazarotene (*Avage*®). These prescriptions are "considered the gold-standard treatments for existing wrinkles," says *Natural Medicines*. Some dermatologists are recommending the off-label use of a less expensive retinoid by using adapalene (*Differin*® Gel) 0.1% daily. The product is marketed and approved OTC only for acne. Its use for skin photoaging is not FDA approved. However, a prescription concentration of 0.3 percent has been shown to be similar in efficacy to *Retin-A*® for photoaging of skin.[16] *Differin*® Gel is about $13 to $16 for a month's supply that will cover the entire face with daily use.

Natural Medicines writes, "Some people think that because tretinoin is a vitamin A derivative, that vitamin A itself might also work. There is no evidence that taking vitamin A supplements orally improves aging skin.

However, there is some evidence that applying vitamin A (as retinol) to the skin might be beneficial."

Natural Medicines also points out, "Retinol preparations are less effective than tretinoin at improving signs of photodamage, so higher concentrations may be needed to achieve comparable effects. One clinical study showed that products containing retinol 1.0% are needed to reduce wrinkles similarly to formulations containing tretinoin 0.1%. Many over-the-counter retinol products contain retinol in lower amounts or do not specify the amount of retinol."

Of note, one of the primary mechanisms for the photoaging treatment by topical retinoids is the production of collagen in collagen-depleted skin.[17] Sun protection will extend the life of natural collagen; however, topical retinoids are known to increase its growth. University of Michigan researchers found that 0.4 percent topical retinol treatment increased the level of type I collagen "in photoaged forearms to levels similar to that of young forearms within four weeks . . . [and] proved the concept that reduced [type I collagen] production in aged skin can be readily restored."[18]

The use of retinoids, adapalene, and retinols can cause mild-to-severe skin reactions in some people and can also increase sensitivity to the sun and ultraviolet (UV) light. Always try a small amount initially.

TOPICAL ALPHA HYDROXY ACIDS (AHAs). As for natural medicines, topical alpha hydroxy acids are very commonly used and are moderately effective. *Natural Medicines* rates them "Likely Safe" and "Likely Effective" for aging skin, advising, "Applying alpha hydroxy acids in a lotion, cream, or solution daily can decrease wrinkles and other signs of aging or photodamage."

AHAs were initially sourced from natural products, such as glycolic acid (from sugar cane), lactic acid (from sour milk), malic acid (from apples), citric acid (from citrus), and tartaric acid (from grapes). However, now the source of the AHAs in most cosmetics is predominantly synthetic.[19] They are a common ingredient in scrubs, lotions, and creams used for wrinkles.

Dr. Griffith notes, "Most moisturizers without AHA gently trap water in the outermost layer of the skin, the stratum corneum, and hydrate those cells. However, moisturizers with added AHA can modify that layer of the skin making it exfoliate and more flexible. It may sting on application, and in conditions of high humidity, it may yield a sticky feel. Many of my patients prefer glycolic acid over lactic acid."

They are also used in higher concentration, short-contact preparations as skin peels, which can help reduce fine wrinkles. *Natural Medicines* rates these products as "moderately effective for improving the signs of aging skin, including reducing wrinkles. They are generally safe and well-tolerated when used short-term and appropriately." However, the use of topical AHAs can cause mild-to-severe skin reactions in some people and can also increase sensitivity to the sun and ultraviolet (UV) light. Always try a small amount initially.

I think of these AHAs based on their concentration:

- High concentrations of 50 to 70 percent are legally used only in physicians' offices.
- Trained cosmetologists use medium concentrations of 20 to 30 percent for light skin peeling.
- Low concentrations of less than 10 to 14 percent are available to the consumer in a variety of products.

Collagen, Vitamin C, Vitamin E, and Other Products

COLLAGEN TYPE I. Adults lose about one percent of the collagen in their skin each year, which contributes to thinning and wrinkling in aging skin. This loss of collagen may be more evident at an earlier age in women, who have lower collagen density in their skin than men. ConsumerLab writes, "Some studies in people suggest that collagen can provide a very modest benefit (10–20 percent improvement) in improving wrinkles by increasing skin volume and elasticity. There is less evidence of a benefit for improving skin hydration and reducing skin roughness." They add, "There are many types of collagen, but the predominant ones in the body are types I, II, and III."

Collagen supplements for the skin typically (but not always) contain type I or type III collagen. ConsumerLab advises, "The best evidence supporting the use of collagen in aging skin is with *Verisol®* (Gelita AG), a collagen peptide made of hydrolyzed, porcine-derived (from pigs) type I collagen." They add that *Verisol®* is "the only ingredient to have been tested in several placebo-controlled clinical trials . . . (showing) a modest improvement in wrinkles after eight weeks and a slight improvement in the appearance of cellulite after six months." *Natural Medicines* rates collagen peptides as "Possibly Safe" and "Possibly Effective" for improving skin hydration and elasticity in older patients and for possibly reducing wrinkles but lists no *Verisol®*-containing products with a NMBER rating higher than 5 out of 10.

ConsumerLab's two "Top Picks" for collagen for skin are "*Trunature®* [Costco®] *Healthy Skin Verisol® Collagen* capsules and *Besha Inc. Collagen Peptides* powder. Both of these products contain collagen peptides (hydrolyzed collagen) from the branded ingredient *Verisol®*." They add, "The products are also reasonably priced, with a daily serving of *Trunature®* (4 capsules) costing 30 cents and providing 2.5 grams of collagen peptides and *Besha* (2 teaspoons) costing 47 cents and providing 2.9 grams of collagen peptides. *Trunature®* is slightly less expensive per gram, but the real deciding factor between the two is whether you prefer to take 4 fairly large capsules daily or mix about 2 teaspoons of powder into your preferred beverage." You can read about *Verisol®* and brittle nails later in this chapter.

ConsumerLab also advises, "Be aware that *Verisol®* is sourced from pigs." If you have dietary restrictions and prefer other sources, ConsumerLab lists products from bovine (cow), chicken, fish, and eggshell products. They add, "The collagen hydrolysates in the powders from *Great Lakes® Gelatin Co.®* and *Vital Proteins®*, for example, are both from bovine hide and are listed as kosher." Labdoor has not rated collagen type I products.

VITAMIN C. A trendy approach to aging skin is to use topical antioxidants to prevent the oxidative damage caused by sun exposure and UV radiation. Vitamin C is perhaps the most common antioxidant included in skincare products. It's available in several active forms. Among them all, L-ascorbic acid is the most biologically active and well-studied.[20] In addition to its antioxidant effects against UV-induced damage, vitamin C may play a role in collagen synthesis and tissue repair.

One recent review concluded, "Topical vitamin C has a wide range of clinical applications, from antiaging and antipigmentary to photoprotective.

Currently, clinical studies on the efficacy of topical formulations of vitamin C remain limited, and the challenge lies in finding the most stable and permeable formulation in achieving the optimal results."[21]

Natural Medicines writes, "Vitamin C is water-soluble, and therefore, taking it orally might not produce high enough concentrations in the skin to be beneficial." However, "Topical preparations containing 5 to 10 percent vitamin C seem to improve the appearance of wrinkled skin." For example, "There is preliminary evidence showing a topical vitamin C formulation (*Cellex-C High-Potency Serum*®, which combines 10 percent vitamin C with tyrosine, zinc, and hyaluronic acid) might help. In three studies, this specific product seems to reduce fine lines, wrinkles, and roughness, and improve skin tone when applied for 12 weeks. In addition, preliminary evidence shows that a 3 percent vitamin C topical preparation applied for 12 weeks might also reduce facial wrinkles."

Natural Medicines adds, "Lots of skin products contain vitamin C, but it might not be obvious after a first glance at the ingredient list. Some products list acerola or rose hip. These are plant materials that contain a high concentration of vitamin C, but there is no reliable evidence that these products are any better than regular vitamin C products." For more information about vitamin C, see the appendix.

VITAMIN E. Vitamin E is also a prevalent antioxidant in skincare products. *Natural Medicines* advises that it is available "both orally and topically. It may improve skin moisture, softness, and smoothness while providing mild protection from ultraviolet sun damage. But so far, there is no reliable clinical evidence that oral or topical vitamin E is helpful for improving signs of aging skin."

However, *Natural Medicines* says, "There is evidence that taking a combination of both vitamin C and vitamin E supplements orally might help in the prevention of photoaging. The most studied dosing is two grams (2000 mg) of vitamin C plus 1,000 IU of vitamin E orally." But they warn that "these high doses might cause adverse effects, including nausea, vomiting, and diarrhea, in some people." In addition, more than 400 IU/day of vitamin E has been linked to increased mortality.[22]

Although an "uncommon phenomena," there are reports of "vitamin E-induced allergic contact dermatitis,"[23] which included several hospitalizations.

Again, I recommend that any time you use a new topical product, you test it on a small area of skin for a few days.

OTHER PRODUCTS. ConsumerLab writes, "Other natural products such as topical alpha-lipoic acid [ALA], topical green tea, coenzyme Q10, lycopene, a chemical derivative of kinetin (furfuryl tetrahydropyranyladenin), and DMAE (dimethylaminoethanol or deanol) are showing promise in clinical research. For example, hyaluronic acid has been evaluated as an oral supplement in combination with other natural medicines (*GliSODin® Skin Nutrients Advanced Anti-Aging Formula*, Isocell North America Inc.), including krill oil, sea buckthorn berry oil, and cacao bean extract." They add, it "moderately decreases wrinkling and photodamage and improves skin moisture and elasticity."

Natural Medicines concludes, "However, it is unclear if these effects are due to hyaluronic acid, other ingredients, or the combination." As a result, they add, "it's too soon to recommend these products as reliable preventive measures or treatments of aging skin."

As to DMAE, ConsumerLab says, "It's showing up in all kinds of facial moisturizers promoted to firm up sagging facial skin. An example is *Reviva® Labs DMAE Firming Fluid, Skin Eternal® Cream*, etc. A one-ounce bottle can cost upwards of $50." I recommend people wait for evidence of safety and effectiveness before purchasing them.

The experts at *Natural Medicines* write, "Patients can spend a *lot* of extra money for products that boast natural ingredients with all sorts of exciting names and scientific-sounding benefits. For now, tell them to save their money until the effects of these ingredients are better understood. Also, explain that more expensive skincare products aren't necessarily more effective. Many cheaper products contain the same ingredients as more expensive brand name products."

An *Atlantic* article with the subtitle "Don't Rub the Money Directly on Your Face," correctly reports the most "natural way" to slow skin aging: "A diet of fresh foods, plenty of water, and eight hours of sleep every night [which affects] how your skin looks. Studies have demonstrated links between all three and physical appearance, and they'll help most people achieve the modest goal of looking totally fine."[24] This is good advice that will also have the rest of your body becoming healthier.

I must give you a warning though. Any of the products mentioned in this chapter can cause mild-to-severe skin reactions in some people and can also increase sensitivity to the sun and ultraviolet (UV) light. I tell my patients to always test topical products on a small area of skin for a day or two before applying it to a larger area. I also warn people to use a sunscreen or wear protective clothing when first trying these products. This increased sensitivity typically resolves within one week of discontinuing treatment.

Brittle Nails

Brittle nails are said to affect approximately 20 percent of the population, and the incidence increases with age. The medical term *onychoschizia* includes splitting, brittle, soft, or thin nails. The American Osteopathic College of Dermatology says, "Other than aging, common causes include frequent wetting and drying, chemical exposure, underlying health or medical problems, stress or trauma, and hormone changes, particularly menopause."[25] Dr. Griffith adds, "Limiting the frequency of fingernail polish removal is helpful. The simplest approach is moisturizers applied to the nails frequently, specifically products containing AHAs."

The most common natural medication recommended for brittle nails is biotin (vitamin B7). ConsumerLab points out, "a small but controlled study among women with brittle nails found that a daily dose of 2.5 mg (2,500 mcg) of biotin for six to nine months increased nail thickness by 25 percent and reduced their tendency to split. Biotin does not, however, further strengthen healthy nails." *Natural Medicines* considers this "Insufficient Evidence" to recommend biotin for brittle nails.

Nevertheless, Marvin M. Lipman, MD, *Consumer Reports*' chief medical adviser, says, "If there are no medical problems causing nail problems, and if nothing shows up after appropriate testing, because we don't have a good blood test to detect biotin deficiency, it might be worthwhile to try a supplement for three months."[26]

This is the approach I have taken with patients in my practice, and, anecdotally, it seems to have been somewhat helpful for people with brittle nails and no discernible medical cause. *Natural Medicines* says it is "Possibly

Safe" and has been "well-tolerated in clinical trials. Relatively high doses up to 300 mg daily for up to 30 months have been taken in some cases without adverse effects."

In a 2020 review, ConsumerLab "Approved" four of five biotin products, advising, "If you want to take biotin for (brittle nails), our 'Top Pick' is *NutraBlast® Hair Skin & Nails*, as it provides 2,500 mcg of biotin per gummy (13 cents)—a bit more expensive than the other 'Approved' products, but the right dose. A less expensive option is *Nature's Life® Biotin 2,500 mcg Hair, Skin and Nails Formula*, which we tested in 2017; each 10-cent capsule provided 2,500 mcg of biotin." USP®-"Verified" *Nature Made® Biotin Adult Gummies*, which at 3,000 mcg (two 1,500 mcg gummies per day) are a slightly higher dose than you need but cost as little as 16 cents a day.

Natural Medicines lists over 110 USP®-"Verified" products containing biotin, with forty of them achieving NMBER ratings of 8 out of 10. Labdoor has "Certified" nine biotin products: four with an "A-plus" rating, four with an "A" rating, and one with an "A-minus" rating. *Nature's Bounty® Biotin* rated "A-plus" and *VitaFusion™ Biotin* rated "A-minus." Both have 1,000 mcg of biotin. The other seven contained 5,000 or 10,000 mcg of biotin,[27] which may be excessive.

There's one last option to consider if the previous suggestions aren't helpful. A small study in women with brittle nails taking *Verisol®* (Gelita AG), 2.5 grams daily for six months, improved overall symptoms of brittle nails. Also, a 12 percent increase in nail growth rate and a 42 percent decrease in broken nail frequency compared to baseline was reported. The study was limited by its small size and lack of a placebo group,[28] so *Natural Medicines* lists it as having "Insufficient Evidence" for effectiveness. However, they do rate it as "Possibly Safe" and "Possibly Effective" for aging skin based upon studies using four to ten grams a day of *Verisol®* for up to twelve weeks. Therefore, it may be worth a try.

Biotin and Lab Tests

ConsumerLab advises, "High doses of biotin (5,000 mcg or more per day) may interfere with certain laboratory tests, so be sure to inform your physician before undergoing tests if you take high doses." Dr. Worthington warns, "There is evidence that even doses as low as 300 mcg daily can interfere with many lab tests."

An FDA Safety Bulletin in 2017 warned, "Patients and physicians may be unaware of biotin interference in laboratory assays." The FDA added, "Be aware that many lab tests, including but not limited to cardiovascular diagnostic tests and hormone tests, that use biotin technology are potentially affected, and incorrect test results may be generated if there is biotin in the patient's specimen."[29]

The American Association for Clinical Chemistry (AACC) Academy, formerly the National Academy of Clinical Biochemistry (NACB), writes, "Most of the published research on biotin interference covers hormone tests, such as parathyroid hormone (PTH), thyroid stimulating hormone (TSH), T4 and T3 tests, as well as tests for troponin (a test for heart damage). However, because biotin is used in so many immunoassays, scientists say it could interfere with many others."[30]

In a 2019 update, the FDA writes that it is "particularly concerned about biotin interference causing a falsely low result for troponin, a clinically important biomarker to aid in the diagnosis of heart attacks, which may lead to a missed diagnosis and potentially serious clinical implications. The FDA continues to receive adverse events reports indicating biotin interference caused falsely low troponin results."[31] The FDA has reported one death that "occurred when a patient taking high doses of biotin had falsely low troponin results from a troponin test known to have interference from biotin. Troponin is a biomarker that helps diagnose heart attacks."[32] Also, researchers have found that even a single dose of biotin can cause a false-positive result for hepatitis B and false-negative results for HIV and hepatitis C blood tests. The researchers advised that biotin from supplements should not be taken for forty-eight hours before blood tests for hepatitis B, hepatitis C, or HIV.[33]

Even though I do not have the space to discuss many other natural medicines advertised for keeping skin and nails young, I've included the ratings for some of the more common ones in the following chart. More detailed information can be obtained from ConsumerLab.com and *Natural Medicines*.

Natural Interventions and Medicines for Aging or Wrinkled Skin and Brittle Nails

Safe / Effective	Likely Safe	Possibly Safe
Effective	★★★★★ **For Skin** • Avoid tobacco • Choose skin-care products with a built-in sun protection factor (SPF) of at least 20 • Eat a nutrient-rich healthy diet • Moisturize your skin • Protect your skin from the sun • Retinoids or retinols	★★★
Likely Effective	★★★★ **For Skin** • Adapalene • Alpha hydroxy acids, topical • Collagen type 1	★★
Possibly Effective	★★★ **For Nails** • Biotin **For Skin** • Hyaluronic acid, topical • L-ascorbic acid, topical • Vitamin C, topical	★ **For Skin** • Alpha-lipoic acid, topical • DHEA (short term) • Gelatin (partially hydro-lyzed collagen) • Pyruvate

Insufficient evidence for safety or effectiveness AND/OR evidence for lack of safety or effectiveness

☹
For Nails
• Collagen type 1
• Multivitamins
For Skin
• Acai
• Acerola
• Acetyl-L-carnitine
• Aloe gel
• Astaxanthin
• Avocado oil
• Beeswax
• Beta-carotene
• Boswellia (Indian frankincense)
• Burdock
• Carrot
• Castor oil

• Chlorophyllin
• Cocoa
• Cocoa butter
• Coconut oil
• Coenzyme Q10
• Collagen hydrolysate
• Collagen type II or III
• Creatine
• Curcumin
• Date palm
• DHEA (long term)
• Dill
• DMAE
• Eggshell membrane hydrolysate
• Emu oil
• Equol
• Glycerol

• Grape	• Papaya
• Grape seed extract	• Peony
• Green tea	• Phenylalanine
• Honey	• Polypodium leucotomos
• Idebenone	• Resveratrol
• Jojoba	• Rose hip
• Kinetin	• Rutin
• Krill oil	• Sea buckthorn
• Lecithin	• Shea butter
• Lycopene	• Soy
• Multivitamins	• Tyrosine
• N-acetyl glucosamine (NAG)	• Vitamin A
• Niacin (vitamin B3)	• Vitamin C
• Niacinamide	• Vitamin E
• Panax ginseng	• Zinc
• Papain	

The recommendations in the chart are based almost entirely on the "Safety and Effectiveness Ratings" contained in *Natural Medicines™* and explained in chapter 4 of this book. They assume the use of high-quality, uncontaminated products and the use of typical doses. Keep in mind that some products are never appropriate for some patients due to concomitant disease states, potential drug interactions, or other clinical factors. Details are available at *Natural Medicines™*.

17

Losing Weight

There are no surprises here! The bottom line is that there is *no* magic bullet; *no* instantly successful pill or potion. There is no natural medicine that is both safe and effective for losing weight. But I'm not here to leave you without hope. There are some possible options to consider.

Overweight and Obesity

Obesity and overweight are conditions that are epidemic in North America, particularly in the US. In 2020, the CDC reported that about seventy percent of US adults were overweight or obese, about forty percent obese, and nearly ten percent severely obese.[1] Obesity is most common in African Americans (48 percent), followed by Hispanics (43 percent), Caucasians (33 percent), and Asians (11 percent).[2]

Body mass index (BMI) is a standardized measure used to diagnose whether you are overweight or obese. There are multiple websites with BMI calculators. You only need to enter your height and weight. It is a useful tool because it is fast and easy. According to the CDC, here's how to interpret your BMI:

- If your BMI is less than 18.5, it falls within the underweight range.
- If your BMI is 18.5 to <25, it falls within the normal range.

- If your BMI is 25.0 to <30, it falls within the overweight range. Some experts say if your BMI is 27.0 to 29.9, it falls into the extreme overweight range.
- If your BMI is 30.0 or higher, it falls within the obese range. [3]

Obesity is frequently subdivided into categories:

- Class 1: BMI of 30 to <35
- Class 2: BMI of 35 to <40
- Class 3: BMI of 40 or higher. This is also called "morbid," "severe," or "extreme" obesity.

However, BMI does not directly measure fat but estimates body fatness based on excess weight. In other words, BMI does not distinguish between weight due to fat, muscle, water/fluids, or bone. As a result, BMI calculations may overestimate body fat in muscular individuals or underestimate body fat in people, especially older people, who have lost muscle. Because of this limitation, many experts recommend using BMI in conjunction with other body-composition tests, including abdominal circumference, skinfold tests, or body fat measured by biometrical impedance. [4]

Consequences of Obesity

Repercussions of the obesity epidemic are enormous.

- The rates of comorbid conditions like type 2 diabetes have sharply increased as obesity raises the risk of diabetes by ten to twenty times. As a result, rates of diabetes have jumped by 60 percent in the last ten years.
- Similarly, obesity is associated with high blood pressure. Evidence suggests that every twenty-pound increase in body weight is associated with a three-point increase in systolic blood pressure and over two points of increase in diastolic blood pressure.
- Obesity is also associated with abnormal lipid levels and elevated levels of inflammatory agents in your bloodstream (fibrinogen and C-reactive protein).

- All of these factors increase the risk of cardiovascular disease events, including coronary heart disease, myocardial infarction, heart failure, and stroke, as well as chronic kidney failure.[5]

Why are so many people overweight or obese? There are several explanations, but the most fundamental reason is that we consume more calories than we burn. Two main reasons for this are increased calorie intake and decreased physical activity.

Other factors that may contribute include genetics and family history. Furthermore, several health conditions (i.e., hypothyroidism or polycystic ovarian syndrome [PCOS]) may cause a person to become overweight. Lastly, some medicines (particularly corticosteroids, antidepressants, or antiepileptic drugs), certain emotional factors (anger, stress, anxiety, depression), smoking cessation, aging, pregnancy, and lack of or poor sleep can contribute to weight gain.

Beware of Weight Loss Claims!

For those who are overweight or obese, multiple medical studies have concluded that the best way to accomplish sustained, healthy weight loss is to aim for a caloric intake that is modestly below daily requirements to create a calorie deficit. For most people, this means lowering total daily calorie intake by 500 to 1,000 calories while adding thirty minutes of exercise at least five days a week. This approach can decrease weight by 5 to 10 percent over three to twelve months. Sadly, most people in the US aren't willing to focus on their nutrition and their exercise.[6]

Approximately 15 percent of US adults have used a weight-loss dietary supplement at some point in their lives; more women (21 percent) report use than men (10 percent). Americans spend about $2.1 billion a year on weight-loss dietary supplements, and one of the top reasons people take dietary supplements is to lose weight. As you'll see, these many millions of Americans are both wasting their money and potentially endangering themselves.

But what about the myriad ads, claims, and testimonials about unbelievable weight loss with supplements? According to the Federal Trade Commission, "Wouldn't it be nice if you could lose weight simply by taking a pill, wearing a patch, or rubbing in a cream? Unfortunately, claims that you can lose weight without changing your habits just aren't true."[7]

Rosario Méndez, an attorney with the FTC, couldn't be clearer: "Ads for weight loss products promise miracles. They might say that the product works for everyone or will let you lose weight permanently. Those claims are lies. Dishonest advertisers will tell you anything to get you to buy their product. They might have images of 'doctors' in their ads and even 'news reports' to make you believe that the product works."

Ms. Méndez adds, "The FTC has investigated, sued, and stopped many companies that made false weight-loss claims in their ads. . . . If you get wooed by a weight-loss ad with wild promises, all you'll lose is your money. And the products might not even be safe."[8]

According to the FTC, "Here are some of the (false) promises from weight loss ads:

- Lose weight without dieting or exercising. (You won't.)
- You don't have to watch what you eat to lose weight. (You do.)
- If you use this product, you'll lose weight permanently. (Wrong.)
- To lose weight, all you have to do is take this pill. (Not true.)
- You can lose 30 pounds in 30 days. (Nope.)
- This product works for everyone. (It doesn't.)
- Lose weight with this patch or cream. (You can't.)

"Here's the truth:

- Any promise of miraculous weight loss is simply untrue.
- There's no magic way to lose weight without a sensible diet and regular exercise.
- No product will let you eat all the food you want and still lose weight.
- Permanent weight loss requires permanent lifestyle changes, so don't trust *any* product that promises once-and-for-all results.
- FDA-approved fat-absorption blockers or appetite suppressants won't result in weight loss on their own; those products are to be taken with a nutrient-dense diet and regular exercise.

- Products promising lightning-fast weight loss are always a scam, and they can ruin your health.

- Even if a product could help some people lose weight in some situations, there's no one-size-fits-all product guaranteed to work for everyone. Everyone's habits and health concerns are unique.

- Nothing you can wear or apply to your skin will cause you to lose weight. Period."[9]

ConsumerLab.com is clear: "There isn't overwhelming evidence that any dietary supplement enables significant, long-term weight loss." The NIH Office of Dietary Supplements writes, "Sellers of (weight loss) supplements might claim that their products help you lose weight by blocking the absorption of fat or carbohydrates, curbing your appetite, or speeding up your metabolism. But there's little scientific evidence that weight-loss supplements work. Many are expensive, some can interact or interfere with medications, and a few might be harmful."[10]

Public health experts from Harvard T.H. Chan School of Public Health in Boston write, "Dietary supplements sold for weight loss . . . are not medically recommended. They have been shown to be ineffective in many cases and pose serious health risks to consumers due to contamination with banned substances, prescription pharmaceuticals, and other dangerous chemicals." The Harvard experts add, "In fact, the FDA has been well aware of this heightened risk for many years." The FDA has issued special warnings in the past "to consumers regarding supplements sold for weight loss, muscle building, and sexual function as being more likely than other supplements to be deceptively marketed and tainted with toxic ingredients."[11]

FDA regulators explain, "Know this: many so-called 'miracle' weight loss supplements and foods (including teas and coffees) don't live up to their claims. Worse, they can cause serious harm."[12] The FDA has discovered hundreds of products that are marketed as dietary supplements but actually contain hidden active ingredients—for example, prescription drugs, unsafe ingredients that were in drugs that have been removed from the market, or compounds that have not been adequately studied in humans.[13]

Near the beginning of this book, I told you about the Dietary Supplement Health and Education Act of 1994 (DSHEA). This federal law makes it the responsibility of the company selling natural medicines to make sure that its products are safe and that any claims made about such products are accurate. Therefore, as the FDA says, "Just because you see a supplement product on a store shelf does not mean it is safe." *Some are dangerous!* Only after safety issues are suspected can the FDA investigate and then, when warranted, take steps to have these products removed from the market.[14] Recent history should be instructive. This list is adapted from Futures Recovery Healthcare:[15]

- Fen-Phen—recalled. Fenfluramine, one of the two active ingredients in the off-label diet drug combination Fen-Phen was recalled in the late 1990s after the drug was linked to cases of heart damage and lung disease. Phentermine, the other primary ingredient in Fen-Phen, is still prescribed in some instances for weight loss but should be used only with a doctor's prescription.
- Ephedra—banned. Once widely sold as an ingredient in diet supplements, ephedra is a Chinese herbal stimulant banned in 2004 because of evidence that its use increased the risk of heart attacks and strokes. In 2005, a lower court ruled that ephedra could be used in small doses. In 2006, a federal appeals court reinstated the FDA's original ban, ruling that ephedra was too dangerous to take as a supplement at any dose.
- *Hydroxycut®*—recalled and banned. *Hydroxycut®* products containing ephedra were banned and recalled in 2009 because of twenty-three reports of liver damage from the drug, one person requiring a liver transplant, and at least one death. In a 2011 report, *CBS News* wrote, "In a normal world a company like [the] maker of the diet supplement Hydroxycut shouldn't exist. Twice its products have killed people. Twice its products have been removed from the market by the FDA. Twice, the company has 'reformulated' the product to replace its active ingredient with a completely different substance. Yet [the company] continues to sell its snake oil, making the same 'clinically proven' claims for each generation

of its product, often with identical wording."[16] *Natural Medicines*™ gives a NMBER® rating of 2 out of 10 for the reformulated product.

- *Meridia®*—withdrawn from the market. Sibutramine, a prescription drug sold as *Meridia®*, prescribed initially as a long-term appetite suppressant and weight-management solution, was voluntarily withdrawn from the market by the manufacturer in 2010 after a clinical study indicated that the drug increased the risk of heart attacks and strokes. In 2018, the FDA announced it had uncovered sixty-eight natural medicines being marketed illegally for weight loss that contained significant amounts of sibutramine.[17]

The FDA warned that it "cannot test all products on the market that contain potentially harmful hidden ingredients. Enforcement actions and consumer advisories for tainted products only cover a small fraction of the tainted over-the-counter products on the market."[18]

The FDA continuously issues public notifications and has issued warning letters, seized products, and criminally prosecuted people responsible for marketing illegal diet products. In addition, the FDA has recalled many tainted weight-loss products and maintains an online list of its public notifications and tainted weight-loss products.[19]

As the FDA concludes, "These deceptive products can harm you!" Unfortunately, as the FDA also warns us, "Hidden ingredients are increasingly becoming a problem in products promoted for weight loss."[20]

Four Natural Medicine Possibilities

According to *Natural Medicines*, there is no herb, vitamin, or dietary supplement (natural medicine) that is "Likely Safe" *or* "Effective" for weight loss. However, there are four worth considering that *may* pan out in the future.

BLOND PSYLLIUM is a water-soluble fiber that has been shown in some preliminary clinical evidence to reduce body weight and appetite in people who are overweight or obese. Unfortunately, there are no long-term studies of its use for weight loss.

Adults may take 3 to 6 grams of psyllium (1 to 2 teaspoons) in or with eight ounces of water two to three times a day (although in studies doses of up to 36 grams a day have been used). ConsumerLab writes:

> Psyllium (such as in *Metamucil®*) may help control hunger. A clinical study (funded by the maker of *Metamucil®*) of 30 healthy adults put on reduced-calorie, low fiber diets found that drinking 6.8 g of psyllium (2 teaspoons) mixed with 1.2 cups of water before breakfast and lunch for three days modestly decreased hunger and desire to eat between meals, as compared to a placebo of matching taste and color. A lower dose (3.4 g) was not as effective, and a higher dose (10.2 g) was no more effective. The specific psyllium product used was *Metamucil® Orange Sugar-Free Fiber Singles* (Procter & Gamble). Mild to moderate gastrointestinal side effects were reported in about 7 percent of people taking 6.8 g psyllium.

Konstyl is a sugar-free (stevia-sweetened) option. ConsumerLab adds, "It's not clear if the same benefits would be seen for a person already consuming greater amounts of fiber from their diet.

A side benefit of blond psyllium, according to *Natural Medicines*, is that 3.4 to 5.1 grams three times a day is "Likely Effective" for lowering cholesterol levels in people with high cholesterol, is "Effective" for improved stool consistency in treating constipation, and is "Possibly Effective" for lowering blood pressure and blood sugar. Psyllium can cause gas and bloating, so many experts recommend starting with lower doses and slowly increasing.

ConsumerLab adds, "Psyllium, a gel-forming viscous soluble fiber, may help control hunger and also improve blood glucose levels and insulin response and modestly lower total and LDL ('bad') cholesterol." Furthermore, *Natural Medicines* warns, "Blond psyllium and other high-fiber products can reduce the absorption of nutrients including calcium, iron, zinc, and vitamin B12 [cobalamin]." They advise health professionals: "For patients taking supplements, including multivitamins, recommend that they take these one hour before or four hours after blond psyllium to avoid this interaction."

While many psyllium-containing supplements list only "psyllium" as an ingredient, there are two types of psyllium: blond psyllium and black psyllium. They come from different plant species. Although both are useful for treating constipation, only blond psyllium has been evaluated for overweight or obese patients.

Natural Medicines lists dozens out of about two hundred products containing blond psyllium that it gives a NMBER rating of 9 out of 10 and about one hundred Canadian-licensed products rated 8 out of 10 or higher. NSF® has "Certified" one psyllium product, but the form of psyllium is not labeled. ConsumerLab and Labdoor have not tested any blond psyllium products. Again, two of the most commercially prominent products are *Metamucil®* and *Konsyl*. For more information about blond psyllium, see the appendix.

CONJUGATED LINOLEIC ACID (CLA). A heavily advertised supplement for weight loss is conjugated linoleic acid (CLA). CLA is primarily found in dairy products and beef. Researchers are evaluating CLA's potential to reduce body fat. Taking 1.8 to 6.8 grams daily seems to decrease body fat mass, increase lean body mass, and reduce waist and hip circumference in some adults. However, CLA does not seem to reduce total body weight or BMI, and there is some concern about its long-term safety.

ConsumerLab concludes, "[CLA] has not been conclusively shown to reduce overall weight." *Natural Medicines* tells health professionals, "Until more is known, advise obese patients against using CLA for weight loss." ConsumerLab did test nine popular CLA products in 2015, and "Approved" seven (a 22 percent failure rate); however, I'd need more information on safety and effectiveness before I could recommend it.

ALPHA-LIPOIC ACID. *Natural Medicines* advises, "Clinical studies and analyses of clinical research show that taking alpha-lipoic acid (ALA) 300–1800 mg daily for 8–48 weeks can modestly reduce body weight by [1–3 pounds] and body mass index . . . when compared with placebo in overweight or obese patients. . . . While these improvements are statistically significant, they may not be clinically meaningful." Again, I'd need more information on safety and effectiveness before I could recommend it.

PHASEOLUS VULGARIS is a starch blocker made from the white kidney bean (*Phaseolus vulgaris*). These products were extensively publicized and sold in the 1970s but removed from the market because the FDA deemed them unproven drugs. Since the passage of DSHEA, starch blockers have been marketed as natural products to avoid the FDA's scrutiny for efficacy.

ConsumerLab says *Phaseolus* "may not be effective for weight loss but may modestly help reduce body fat at doses ranging from 445 mg to 3,000 mg per day." Some studies have evaluated *Phaseolus vulgaris* extract combined with other ingredients (garcinia extract, inulin from chicory root, or elemental chromium) and found the combination products modestly reduced weight, BMI, and percent body fat in obese individuals. *Phaseolus* is generally safe in short-term clinical studies with the most commonly reported side effect being mild gastrointestinal symptoms.[21]

ConsumerLab has "Approved" one *Phaseolus* product, *Rock Star™ Skinny Gal™ Thermogenic*. Although this product claimed "No caffeine," ConsumerLab found 51.6 mg per serving with a cost of "50 cents per serving." *Natural Medicines* lists no US products (out of over five hundred) that are NMBER rated at 8 out of 10 or higher. I would need more data on effectiveness, safety, and quality to recommend any *Phaseolus* product.

The Bottom Line: What Actually Works!

For my patients who are overweight or obese, I recommend the following:

1. *Nutrition!* It's not just a cliché: "A moment on the lips means a lifetime on the hips," or as my wife's family says, "Put it on the lips, wear it on the hips!" Scientists have proven that "even short periods of bingeing on junk food can leave the body more prone to gain weight for years to come."[22] So what's the best nutrition plan for weight loss? Everyone has an opinion, but what do the experts say? My favorite answer to this question comes from annual ratings of diets from *US News and World Reports*. The editors convene "a panel of food and health experts to rank 35 diets on a variety of measures," such as "the diet's ability to help a person lose weight in the short and long term."

   What did they recommend in their 2020 report? In the "Best Weight-Loss Diets" category, they rank the WW (Weight Watchers) diet #1, the Vegan diet #2, and the Volumetrics diet #3. In the

"Best Fast Weight Loss" category, they rate the HMR Program #1, the Optavia diet #2, and the Atkins diet #3. Finally, in the "Best Commercial Diet Plans" category, *US News* recommends the WW (Weight Watchers) diet #1, the Jenny Craig diet #2, and the Nutritarian diet #3. You can read much more about each of them at tinyurl.com/v6ydcfx.

Also, for the third consecutive year, the Mediterranean diet ranked #1 as the "Best Diet Overall." (Read more about it in chapter 8, "Cholesterol and Dyslipidemia.")

If you can afford it, I'd start with one of the top commercial plans, and then once you are successful, I'd recommend transitioning to the Mediterranean diet.

Dr. Worthington writes, "We have a number of diet monographs on our site, and many of them show short-term benefit for weight loss. However, it's hard to say which diet is best to recommend. Overall, following any one specific diet is probably less important than focusing on overall calorie reduction. Ensuring that a diet promotes moderation AND meets individual preferences is the best way to ensure that a diet strategy will lead to long-term adherence and weight loss maintenance."

The CDC adds, "The key to achieving and maintaining a healthy weight isn't about short-term dietary changes. It's about a lifestyle that includes healthy eating, regular physical activity, and balancing the number of calories you consume with the number of calories your body uses."[23]

2. *Movement!* I recommend walking because it is simple. Aim for 150 minutes a week. That's just 30 minutes a day, five days a week. And, your 30 minutes doesn't have to be in one session. The CDC says three 10-minute sessions have the same healthful benefits.[24]

   According to the most recent physical activity guidelines published in *JAMA*, "Even two minutes of any physical activity—taking the stairs, walking the dog, or carrying out the trash—can add up to significant health benefits, such as improved blood pressure, enhanced brain function, reduced risk of cancer, and weight loss."[25]

However, as preventive medicine expert Thomas McKnight, MD, MPH, says, "It's easy for patients to take in more calories by eating than they are burning with exercise. The elbow is more powerful than the knees, in that sense."[26]

3. *Restful sleep!* This one is a surprise to most of my patients. Yet, as WebMD writes, "Catching enough ZZZs is almost as important as exercise or nutrition if you're looking to lose weight. Studies link a lack of sleep to feeling hungrier and gaining weight. When you skimp on shut-eye, you're more likely to eat bigger portions, crave high-carb foods, and choose fatty snacks. Plus, chances are you'll be too tired to work out—a double whammy. Try to aim for 7 to 8 hours per night."[27] This is due to sleep's impact on two essential hunger hormones, ghrelin and leptin. I tell my patients, "Ghrelin gives you a Greater appetite, while Leptin gives you Less appetite. When you do not get adequate sleep, the body makes more ghrelin and less leptin, leaving you hungry and increasing your appetite."[28]

If you can't follow these three recommendations or they don't work for you, don't turn to false promises, unnecessary expense, and the potential danger of natural medicines for weight loss. Dr. Worthington warns, "Weight loss supplements are one of the top three classes of supplements that are tainted with unlisted drugs." Instead, turn to your family physician to discuss adding either an over-the-counter or a prescription anti-obesity drug to use along with items number 1 through 3 above.

If you're overweight or obese, there *is* hope in these recommendations. The National Weight Control Registry housed at Brown School of Medicine is a research study that includes people eighteen years or older who have lost at least thirty pounds of weight and kept it off for at least one year. There are currently over ten thousand members enrolled in the study, making it perhaps the most extensive study of weight loss ever conducted. Members complete annual questionnaires about their current weight, diet, and exercise habits and behavioral strategies for weight loss maintenance.[29]

The research has shown that those registered lost weight by a wide variety of methods. However, 98 percent modified their food intake, while 94 percent increased their exercise. After losing weight, almost all the participants ate breakfast and weighed themselves regularly, most commonly once per week. About 45 percent lost weight on their own, while 55 percent received help from some type of program. Also, the majority watched less TV than average and engaged in about sixty minutes per day of moderate-intensity physical activity, or the equivalent.[30] As Dr. McKnight says, "It's not easy, but it's doable!"

Although I do not have the space to discuss the many other natural medicines that are being sold for weight loss, I've included ratings of the more common ones in the following chart. More detailed information is available from ConsumerLab.com and *Natural Medicines*.

Natural Interventions and Medications for Weight Loss, Overweight, and Obesity

Safe / Effective	Likely Safe	Possibly Safe
Effective	★★★★★ • Diet high in fruits and vegetables • Diet of nutrient-dense food • Exercise • Restful sleep	★★★
Likely Effective	★★★★ • Volumetrics diet	★★
Possibly Effective	★★★ • Atkins diet • Blond psyllium • Caffeine • DASH diet • Fiber-rich diet • Flaxseed • Ketogenic diet (short term) • Vegan diet • Vegetarian diet • Whey protein	★ • Agar • Aloe • Alpha-lipoic acid • Cissus quadrangularis • Conjugated linoleic acid (CLA) • Diacylglycerol • Grapefruit • Inulin (short term) • Mangosteen • Paleo diet • Phaseolus vulgaris • Pyruvate • Resveratrol

Insufficient evidence for safety or effectiveness AND/OR evidence for lack of safety or effectiveness

⊗

- 1-3 DMAA
- 5-HTP
- 7-keto-DHEA
- Acacia
- Acupressure
- Acupuncture
- Alpha hydroxy acids (AHAs)
- Anti-inflammatory diet
- Apple
- Apple cider vinegar
- Apple polyphenols
- Aristolochia
- Astragalus
- Avocado
- Avocado soy unsaponifiables (ASU)
- Banana
- Barley
- Berberine
- Beta-glucans
- Beta-hydroxybutyrate (BHB)
- Betaine anhydrous
- Bifidobacteria
- Bilberry
- Bitter orange
- Black psyllium
- Black seed
- Black tea
- Blue-green algae
- Calcium
- Canola oil
- Capsicum
- Caralluma
- Caraway
- Carnosine
- Carob
- Casein protein
- Cassia cinnamon
- Ceylon cinnamon
- Cha de bugre
- Chia
- Chitosan
- Chokeberry
- Chromium
- Cinnamomum burmannii
- Cocoa
- Coconut oil
- Coffee
- Coleus
- Collagen peptides
- Damiana
- DHEA
- DMAA
- Docosahexaenoic acid (DHA)
- Elderberry
- Ephedra
- Evening primrose
- Fenugreek
- Fish oil
- Flaxseed oil
- Fucus vesiculosus
- Galacto-oligosaccharides (GOS)
- Garcinia
- Garlic
- Ginger
- Glucomannan
- Glutamine
- Glycerol
- Glycomacropeptide
- Goji
- Grape
- Green coffee
- Green coffee extract
- Green tea
- Griffonia simplicifolia
- Guarana
- Guar gum
- Guggul
- Gymnema
- Hazelnut
- HCG diet
- Hesperidin
- Hibiscus
- Holy basil
- Hoodia
- Hydroxycitric acid (HCA)
- Hydroxymethylbutyrate (HMB)
- Hypnotherapy
- Irvingia gabonensis
- Jiaogulan
- Kefir
- Kola nut

- Kudzu
- Lactobacillus
- L-arginine
- L-carnitine
- Licorice
- Lupin
- Magnolia
- Manchurian thorn
- Manganese
- Medium chain triglycerides (MCTs)
- Mindfulness
- Moringa
- Moxibustion
- Nicotinamide riboside
- Olive
- Onion
- Oolong tea
- Organic food
- Ornish diet
- Pear
- Phellodendron
- Phenylalanine
- Plant sterols
- Pomegranate
- Prenatal vitamins
- Prickly pear cactus
- Probiotics
- Quinoa
- Raspberry ketone
- Rehmannia
- Rhubarb
- Rose hip
- Royal jelly
- Sea buckthorn
- Slim-Fast diet
- Soy
- St. John's wort
- Sweet almond
- Sweet orange
- Tai chi
- Tiratricol
- Tyrosine
- Usnea
- Vitamin D
- Willow bark
- Yerba maté
- Yogurt
- Yohimbe

Most of the recommendations in the chart are based on the "Safety and Effectiveness Ratings" contained in *Natural Medicines™* and explained in chapter 4 of this book. They assume the use of high-quality, uncontaminated products and the use of typical doses. Keep in mind that some products are never appropriate for some patients due to concomitant disease states, potential drug interactions, or other clinical factors. Details are available at *Natural Medicines™*.

APPENDIX

Safety and Effectiveness for Each Natural Medicine or Intervention in This Book

As I mentioned earlier in this book, I've evaluated almost 1,300 natural medicines or interventions covering about 550 conditions or indications. It's actually quite shocking to see how few can be recommended—only 410 out of 1,298 (about 32 percent). In point of fact, most (888 or about 67 percent) don't have evidence of safety and/or effectiveness. In other words, they would not only be a waste of time and money but could also be dangerous.

Of the ~1,300 natural medicines and interventions I evaluated for ~550 conditions/indications

★★★★★	83	6%	150	11%
★★★★	67	5%		
★★★	88	7%	260	22%
★★	69	5%		
★	103	10%		
☹	888	67%	888	67%

KEY

★★★★★	I recommend considering in almost all cases (Effective and Likely Safe)
★★★★	I recommend in many to most cases (Likely Effective & Likely Safe)
★★★	I recommend in some cases (Effective & Possibly Safe)
★★	I recommend in a few cases (Likely Effective & Possibly Safe OR Possibly Effective & Possibly Safe)
★	I recommend in unusual cases (Possibly Effective & Possibly Safe)
⊗	I recommend against using (Insufficient Evidence, Possibly Ineffective, Possibly Unsafe, Ineffective, or Unsafe)

Acknowledgments

For over twenty years, I have used the resources from two organizations, ConsumerLab.com and *Natural Medicines™*, while caring for patients day-to-day and in my lay and professional writing, media interviews, and presentations. I'm most grateful to each for allowing me access to and permission to quote from and adapt some of their respective treasure troves of remarkably complete and amazingly applicable information.

For any person or organization interested in continually updated, nonbiased, evidence-based, well-referenced, and clinically trustworthy information on any natural medicine or alternative therapy, or for any healthcare institution or health professional who is or will be making recommendations to patients or consumers about any herb, vitamin, or supplement, subscriptions to both of these organizations come with my highest recommendation.

Thanks to Tod Cooperman, MD, president, founder, and editor-in-chief of ConsumerLab.com and Mark L. Anderson, PhD, vice president for research for ConsumerLab.com for freely offering me their expertise, critique, research, and resources for this book. Dr. Cooperman, although an incredibly busy man, personally reviewed each chapter of the book for accuracy. Thanks, Tod. It's a better book because of you and ConsumerLab.com.

I'm also extremely grateful for the expertise and assistance of TRC Healthcare and for their extensive library of resources, which includes *Hospital Pharmacist's Letter™*, *Hospital Pharmacy Technician's Letter™*, *Prescriber's Letter™*, *Pharmacist's Letter™*, *Pharmacy Technician's*

Letter™, and *Natural Medicines*™ (formerly the *Natural Medicines Comprehensive Database*). Thanks to Joshua Conrad, PharmD, vice president of editorial and content, and most especially to Amanda Brownlie, content and digital marketing manager, and Meredith Worthington, PhD, former director and senior editor for *Natural Medicines*. Amanda and Meredith are tremendously talented women whose schedules were already filled to the brim, yet who took an incredible amount of their professional time to review every chapter, chart, and recommendation of this book. They unselfishly contributed their considerable professional expertise to make this a far more useful and complete book than I ever could have imagined. They allowed me to freely utilize their mammoth collection of brand reviews, guidelines, recommendations, and NMBER® ratings as well as their extensive professional and patient monographs. Thanks, Amanda and Meredith. You're amazing.

I'm grateful for another devoted group of practicing health professionals who critically reviewed the manuscript to assure that it was up to date, trustworthy, and medically reliable. They include Sandra L. Argenio, MD; Tim Dornemann, EdD, CES, PES, CSCS; Sherri Flynt, MPH, RD, LD; Steve Foley, MD, FACOG; Robert Griffith, MD, FAAD; Douglas Henley, MD, FAAFP; Susan Henriksen, MD, FAAFP; Sarah Jones, MD, FAAFP; Dilip Joseph, MD, MPH; Sam Kammerzell, DO; Tom Kintinar, MD, FAAFP; Huy Luu, MD, FAAFP; Tom McKnight, MD, MPH, MDiv; Dale Michaels, MD, FAAFP; Shawn Morehead, MD, FAAFP; Cherec Morrison, MD; Mary Anne Nelson, MD, FAAFP; Dan Ostergaard, MD, FAAFP; Cathie Scarborough, MD, FAAFP, and David S. Seres, MD, ScM, PNS, FASPEN.

The Centers for Disease Control and Prevention and the National Institutes of Health (especially the NIH National Center for Complementary and Integrative Health, National Institute on Aging, and Office of Dietary Supplements) provided excellent information and assistance, and allowed me to freely use their information, advice, and recommendations.

Thanks also to Don Jones of Studio Commercial Photography for allowing me to use a portrait he took of me. You can see his amazing work at tinyurl.com/y37xk5ou. I'm grateful to my agent, Greg Johnson, founder and president of WordServe Literary, who worked so diligently to find a home for this book.

Acknowledgments

I am fortunate to have the opportunity to work with Revell, a division of Baker Publishing Group, to make this handbook available to you. A special thanks to my dear friend Cindy Lambert, who was my first editor and has edited almost all of my health books and memoirs through the years. Cindy, I love and admire you deeply. I appreciate so much Vicki Crumpton, executive editor at Revell, and Gisèle Mix, project editor, who improved the original manuscript in myriad ways. Thanks to Gayle Raymer, art director at Baker Publishing Group, and her team for their fabulous work on the front and back covers, as well as Wendy Wetzel, associate marketing manager at Revell and her team, including Janelle Wiesen. I appreciate the efforts of Erin Bartels, trade catalog manager.

I especially appreciate the support of my friend of sixty-four years, my best friend of fifty-two years, and my wife of nearly forty-eight years, Barb Larimore, for her endless love, support, prayers, and wonderful and wise editing.

Walter L. Larimore, MD
Colorado Springs, CO
November 2020

Other Resources
from Walt Larimore, MD

Health Books

Alternative Medicine: The Options, the Claims, the Evidence, How to Choose Wisely (with Dónal O'Mathúna)

Fit over 50: Make Simple Choices Today for a Healthier, Happier You (with Phillip Bishop)

God's Design for the Highly Healthy Child (with Stephen and Amanda Sorenson)

God's Design for the Highly Healthy Person (with Traci Mullins)

God's Design for the Highly Healthy Teen (with Mike Yorkey)

The Highly Healthy Child (with Traci Mullins)

Lintball Leo's Not-So-Stupid Questions about Your Body (with John Riddle)

SuperSized Kids: How to Rescue Your Child from the Obesity Threat (with Sherri Flynt and Steve Halliday)

10 Essentials of Highly Healthy People: Becoming and Staying Highly Healthy

The Ultimate Girls' Body Book: Not-So-Silly Questions about Your Body (with Amaryllis Sánchez Wohlever)

The Ultimate Guys' Body Book: Not-So-Stupid Questions about Your Body

Why ADHD Doesn't Mean Disaster (with Dennis Swanburg and Diane Passno)

Memoirs from My Practice

The Best Medicine: Tales of Humor and Hope from a Small-Town Doctor

The Best Gift: Tales of a Small-Town Doctor Learning Life's Greatest Lessons (Coming in October 2021)

Bryson City Tales: Stories of a Doctor's First Year of Practice in the Smoky Mountains

Bryson City Seasons: More Tales of a Doctor's Practice in the Smoky Mountains

Bryson City Secrets: Even More Tales of a Small-Town Doctor in the Smoky Mountains

Web Resources

www.DrWalt.com
www.DrWalt.com/blog
www.Devotional.DrWalt.com

Notes

Disclaimer

1. https://tinyurl.com

Introduction

• ConsumerLab.com quotes are from:

   1. "About ConsumerLab.com," tinyurl
      .com/yck2tbp.
   2. "ConsumerLab.com Annual Vitamin &
      Supplement Users Survey and Survey
      Report," tinyurl.com/rndadmz.
   3. "How to Read a ConsumerLab.com
      Approved Quality Product Seal,"
      tinyurl.com/uboam2r.
   4. "Vitamin C Supplements Review,"
      last updated July 1, 2020, tinyurl
      .com/y3g8vc5t.

• *Natural Medicines*™ quotes are from:

   1. "Editorial Principles and Process,"
      trchealthcare.com.

• Quotes from Meredith Worthington, PhD,
  are from an email communication, October 15, 2019.

   1. tinyurl.com/sduqqbo
   2. tinyurl.com/sduqqbo
   3. tinyurl.com/u9aqxor

**Chapter 1 Natural Medicines Are
Popular**

• ConsumerLab.com quotes are from:

   1. "Collagen and Magnesium
      Rise in Popularity, as Fish Oil
      and Curcumin Dip in Latest
      ConsumerLab Survey of Supplement
      Users," February 29, 2020, tinyurl
      .com/vtvdq4o.
   1. tinyurl.com/yc5t22zj
   2. tinyurl.com/y2uow5cg
   3. tinyurl.com/yyfsfjk6
   4. tinyurl.com/yyfsfjk6
   5. tinyurl.com/y4g3g7lm
   6. tinyurl.com/y62rtqwv
   7. tinyurl.com/yc5t22zj
   8. tinyurl.com/y3oathrb
   9. tinyurl.com/y6y4r568
   10. tinyurl.com/y6y4r568
   11. tinyurl.com/y6y4r568
   12. tinyurl.com/yxm9p6tt
   13. tinyurl.com/rwcm9lr
   14. tinyurl.com/yawtm4n3
   15. tinyurl.com/y2ulyyoa
   16. tinyurl.com/y6y4r568

Chapter 2 Natural Medicines Are Problematic

• ConsumerLab.com and Tod Cooperman, MD, quotes are from:

1. "Dr. Tod Cooperman's Testimony to Senate Special Committee on Aging, Subcommittee on Dietary Supplements," May 26, 2010, tinyurl.com/y4b4jjlb.
2. "FDA Finds Problems at 52% of Supplement Manufacturing Sites in US and 42% Abroad," March 13, 2020, tinyurl.com/vkhr2vu.

• *Natural Medicines*™ quotes are from:

1. "Are Dietary Supplements Regulated?," News, June 2019.
2. "FDA Clamps Down on Supplement Claims for Alzheimer's Disease," News, April 2019.
3. "Supplement-Related Calls to Poison Control Centers on the Rise," News, March 2019.

• Quotes from Meredith Worthington, PhD, are from an email communication, July 22, 2019.

1. tinyurl.com/y264xawr
2. tinyurl.com/tyrxluz
3. tinyurl.com/yckhbc5u
4. tinyurl.com/yckhbc5u
5. tinyurl.com/wmbpkma
6. tinyurl.com/y6ss5djm
7. tinyurl.com/y264xawr
8. tinyurl.com/y6dbwpp9
9. tinyurl.com/wtelpgl
10. tinyurl.com/yymxhnax
11. tinyurl.com/yymxhnax
12. tinyurl.com/yymxhnax
13. tinyurl.com/unsdgtb
14. tinyurl.com/yb3j43uy
15. tinyurl.com/y27wxb8c
16. tinyurl.com/y264xawr
17. tinyurl.com/y2ulyyoa
18. tinyurl.com/wouck7h
19. tinyurl.com/yxea8txs
20. tinyurl.com/suo2nhz
21. tinyurl.com/y2ulyyoa
22. tinyurl.com/y53hn6hz
23. tinyurl.com/y8v4pyyd
24. tinyurl.com/y6k6c5ad
25. tinyurl.com/y7evl7b8
26. tinyurl.com/y6weu2on
27. tinyurl.com/nhbozqz
28. tinyurl.com/y4euh8pn
29. tinyurl.com/q6rgxak
30. tinyurl.com/y3fyrv39
31. tinyurl.com/y5jnept6
32. tinyurl.com/yyc44hjw
33. tinyurl.com/y53hn6hz
34. tinyurl.com/uk8zjrk
35. tinyurl.com/y29c2muc

Chapter 3 What's More Effective Than *Any* Natural Medicine?

1. tinyurl.com/yyp2fld8
2. tinyurl.com/yyp2fld8
3. tinyurl.com/v9vlceo
4. tinyurl.com/v9vlceo
5. tinyurl.com/twupd49
6. tinyurl.com/auqchza
7. tinyurl.com/bejyhq3
8. tinyurl.com/y88wztaq

Chapter 4 Safety and Effectiveness Ratings

• *Natural Medicines*™ quotes are from:

1. "Editorial Principles and Process," trchealthcare.com.

Chapter 5 An Overall Approach to Wellness and Multivitamins

• ConsumerLab.com quotes are from:

1. "Multivitamin and Multimineral Supplements Review," Product Reviews, last updated August 21, 2020, tinyurl.com/yyz4kzhb.

• *Natural Medicines*™ quotes are from:

1. "Multivitamins for Heart Disease: Lifesaver or Waste of Money?," News, September 2018.
2. "Multivitamins," Professional Monograph, last updated May 7, 2020.

• Quotes from Meredith Worthington, PhD, are from email communications, 2019–2020.

1. tinyurl.com/qjpyyfa
2. tinyurl.com/y5sludea
3. tinyurl.com/y5sludea
4. tinyurl.com/v9geg7y
5. tinyurl.com/wn7bj2x
6. tinyurl.com/hyr2kok
7. tinyurl.com/ybt5mmfj
8. tinyurl.com/m5oopoj
9. tinyurl.com/t5ngsoh
10. tinyurl.com/vdahfl3
11. tinyurl.com/yyp2fld8
12. tinyurl.com/ubfkxek
13. tinyurl.com/ubfkxek
14. tinyurl.com/ubfkxek
15. tinyurl.com/ycmk5hfx
16. tinyurl.com/ycmk5hfx
17. tinyurl.com/ybadn9cl
18. tinyurl.com/y7tntsc3
19. tinyurl.com/wrxx892
20. tinyurl.com/rb75r5s
21. 1 Timothy 4:8
22. 3 John 1:2
23. tinyurl.com/y5gqx4oe
24. tinyurl.com/y6y4r568
25. tinyurl.com/yx7ontk6
26. tinyurl.com/yx7ontk6
27. tinyurl.com/y62rtqwv
28. tinyurl.com/tcgqf75
29. tinyurl.com/y2t7vue8
30. tinyurl.com/y4625p3c
31. tinyurl.com/sza9qqp
32. tinyurl.com/y3l32luy
33. tinyurl.com/y47z8ceq
34. tinyurl.com/y3l32luy
35. tinyurl.com/y5jdplmg
36. tinyurl.com/y6yhxzd2
37. tinyurl.com/y3bstsk2
38. tinyurl.com/y2pf9t72; tinyurl.com/yygps676
39. tinyurl.com/y4np7ws2
40. tinyurl.com/y2m7g6bp
41. tinyurl.com/ya25ceqe
42. tinyurl.com/yxavklcr
43. tinyurl.com/y4auzo2d
44. tinyurl.com/ltu8ea6
45. tinyurl.com/y48negqu
46. tinyurl.com/y2m62cp3
47. tinyurl.com/y4vxvxh6
48. tinyurl.com/3xayfy

Chapter 6 Brain Health—Part 1

• ConsumerLab.com quotes are from:

1. "Ginkgo (Ginkgo Biloba) Supplements Review," Product Review, last updated November 16, 2019, tinyurl.com/qu9oe25.
2. "Huperzine A Supplements Review," Product Review, last updated February 4, 2020, tinyurl.com /sahnwck.

• *Natural Medicines*™ quotes are from:

1. "Beta-Carotene," Professional Monograph, last updated March 16, 2020.
2. "Copper," Professional Monograph, last updated March 10, 2020.
3. "Fish Oil," Professional Monograph, last updated September 30, 2020.
4. "Folic Acid," Professional Monograph, last updated August 18, 2020.
5. "Huperzine A," Professional Monograph, last updated January 15, 2020.
6. "Is Your Ginkgo Supplement Tainted?," News, December 2019.
7. "Natural Medicines in Geriatric Patients," Clinical Management Series, July 1, 2019.
8. "Selenium," Professional Monograph, last updated July 28, 2020.
9. "Vitamin B6," Professional Monograph, last updated September 18, 2020.
10. "Vitamin B12," Professional Monograph, last updated September 18, 2020.
11. "Vitamin D," Professional Monograph, last updated August 28, 2020.
12. "Vitamin E," Professional Monograph, last updated July 24, 2020.

13. "Zinc," Professional Monograph, last updated August 19, 2020.

• Quote from Meredith Worthington, PhD, is from an email communication, October 15, 2019.

1. tinyurl.com/y4j5ywsx
2. tinyurl.com/wauvwpm
3. tinyurl.com/sow9q9e
4. tinyurl.com/y2cao3t5
5. tinyurl.com/tvfy65n
6. tinyurl.com/rhp8x6r
7. tinyurl.com/y3z7dls7
8. tinyurl.com/tjptbq3
9. tinyurl.com/t7lwkbm
10. tinyurl.com/y3nef7ut
11. tinyurl.com/vfa7wmp
12. tinyurl.com/szpauo7
13. tinyurl.com/y3rum2n6
14. tinyurl.com/re2tq7d
15. tinyurl.com/t2hgbya
16. tinyurl.com/tjptbq3
17. tinyurl.com/szpauo7
18. tinyurl.com/sz8edhs
19. tinyurl.com/wauvwpm
20. tinyurl.com/tuqhq59
21. tinyurl.com/v9vlceo
22. tinyurl.com/y2ncrxst
23. tinyurl.com/tklzwca
24. tinyurl.com/yykk3pnt
25. tinyurl.com/v9vlceo
26. tinyurl.com/y24t7ua3
27. tinyurl.com/uqz3swl
28. tinyurl.com/y2ujgxen
29. tinyurl.com/yyp2fld8
30. tinyurl.com/usufq8d
31. tinyurl.com/y3z7dls7
32. tinyurl.com/y3nef7ut
33. tinyurl.com/y3rum2n6
34. tinyurl.com/swz4k53
35. tinyurl.com/y3rum2n6
36. tinyurl.com/y3rum2n6
37. tinyurl.com/y37aesk7
38. tinyurl.com/y3rum2n6
39. tinyurl.com/swz4k53
40. tinyurl.com/szpauo7
41. November 2020 issues of *Pharmacist's Letter* and *Prescriber's Letter*, tinyurl.com/yydon6qr.
42. tinyurl.com/s8gmk8g
43. tinyurl.com/uw8ymls
44. tinyurl.com/t2hgbya
45. tinyurl.com/y39dqh7q
46. tinyurl.com/y5xauk3y
47. tinyurl.com/s8gmk8g
48. tinyurl.com/t5gqwq8
49. tinyurl.com/szpauo7
50. tinyurl.com/szpauo7

Chapter 7 Brain Health—Part 2

• ConsumerLab.com quotes are from:

1. "'Brain Boosting' Supplements Were Promoted with Non-Existent Clinical Studies," Recalls and Warnings, April 23, 2019, tinyurl.com/tngb7ze.
2. "Brain Bright for Memory?," ConsumerLab.com Answers, tinyurl.com/vksosjx.
3. "Does Fisetin Really Help Improve Memory?," ConsumerLab.com Answers, tinyurl.com/tnr4w8r.
4. "Does Prevagen Really Improve Memory?," ConsumerLab.com Answers, tinyurl.com/t8pxz5y.
5. "Pomegranate Juice and Supplements Review Article," Product Review, last updated February 1, 2020, tinyurl.com/sdabzq4.

• *Natural Medicines*™ quotes are from:

1. "Brain Bright by BioTrust Nutrition," Commercial Products.
2. "Fisetin With Novusetin by Doctor's Best," Commercial Products.
3. "Neuriva Original by Schiff Neuriva," Commercial Products.
4. "Neuriva Plus by Schiff Neuriva," Commercial Products.
5. "New Guidelines: Dementia Prevention," News, July 2019.
6. "Novusetin by Cyvex Nutrition, Inc.," Commercial Products.
7. "Phenibut," Product Monograph, last updated November 14, 2019.
8. "Prevagen by Quincy Bioscience," Commercial Products.

9. "Prevagen Remains Popular Despite No Supportive Evidence," News, October 2020.
10. "Supplements for Brain Health?," News, November 2019.
1. tinyurl.com/szpauo7
2. tinyurl.com/rwgtl3e
3. tinyurl.com/tyvlesz
4. tinyurl.com/vaqbzex
5. tinyurl.com/vzqk636
6. tinyurl.com/y8qylvn5
7. tinyurl.com/y2ooxuny
8. tinyurl.com/vtu7sls
9. tinyurl.com/vtu7sls
10. tinyurl.com/y326pgos
11. tinyurl.com/y6k6c5ad
12. tinyurl.com/rvxqpzf
13. tinyurl.com/v5l3c8u
14. tinyurl.com/s8gmk8g
15. tinyurl.com/s8gmk8g
16. tinyurl.com/t2hgbya
17. tinyurl.com/t2hgbya
18. tinyurl.com/t2hgbya
19. tinyurl.com/t2hgbya
20. tinyurl.com/t2hgbya
21. tinyurl.com/t2hgbya
22. tinyurl.com/usufq8d
23. tinyurl.com/uzbsdfb
24. tinyurl.com/tlgtquv
25. tinyurl.com/usufq8d
26. tinyurl.com/tlgtquv
27. tinyurl.com/y26n9gc4; tinyurl.com/y37t9z5y
28. tinyurl.com/tlgtquv
29. tinyurl.com/usufq8d
30. tinyurl.com/y3nef7ut
31. tinyurl.com/s8gmk8g
32. tinyurl.com/uzephac
33. tinyurl.com/uuauyfa
34. tinyurl.com/s8gmk8g
35. tinyurl.com/yx36nlcc
36. tinyurl.com/wmd3vub
37. tinyurl.com/wmd3vub
38. tinyurl.com/wmd3vub

Chapter 8 Cholesterol and Dyslipidemia

• ConsumerLab.com quotes are from:
1. "Cholesterol-Lowering Supplements Review (Sterols/Stanols and Policosanol)," Product Reviews, initial post April 20, 2019, tinyurl.com/vfrq8wb.
2. "Fish Oil and Omega-3 and -7 Supplements Review (Including Krill, Algae, Calamari, and Sea Buckthorn)," Product Reviews, last updated September 25, 2020, tinyurl.com/3lud98j.
3. "Fish Oil Supplements vs. Prescription Vascepa," ConsumerLab.com Answers, November 13, 2018, tinyurl.com/wdt3t2a.
4. "Red Yeast Rice Supplements Review," Product Reviews, last updated February 8, 2020, tinyurl.com/ssyrr7o.

• *Natural Medicines*™ quotes are from:
1. "Benecol Smart Chews by McNeil Consumer Healthcare," Commercial Products.
2. "Benecol Softgels by McNeil Consumer Healthcare," Commercial Products.
3. "DASH Diet," Professional Monograph, last updated April 8, 2020.
4. "Dietary and Lifestyle Interventions for Overweight and Obesity," Clinical Management Series, December 1, 2019.
5. "Mediterranean Diet," Professional Monograph, last updated February 24, 2020.
6. "Natural Medicines in the Clinical Management of Hyperlipidemia," Clinical Management Series, November 1, 2019.
7. "Red Yeast Rice," Professional Monograph, last updated July 24, 2020.
8. "Sitostanol," Professional Monograph, last updated December 14, 2018.
1. tinyurl.com/y6e3zcry
2. tinyurl.com/yxp9gprb
3. tinyurl.com/y55a5anv
4. tinyurl.com/rsvby39

5. tinyurl.com/ydddc8rl
6. tinyurl.com/ycfrux8b
7. tinyurl.com/yazwknqu
8. tinyurl.com/yazwknqu
9. tinyurl.com/yazwknqu
10. tinyurl.com/t8elexo
11. tinyurl.com/y55a5anv
12. tinyurl.com/wc4gr2h
13. tinyurl.com/ybhdqzly
14. tinyurl.com/ybhdqzly
15. tinyurl.com/y55a5anv
16. tinyurl.com/ybybkphm
17. tinyurl.com/ycthmasb
18. tinyurl.com/rys94va
19. tinyurl.com/v5yz8sj
20. tinyurl.com/tmnwm4a
21. tinyurl.com/wbwhwe4
22. tinyurl.com/wpfu2hl
23. tinyurl.com/yaw7r5f7
24. tinyurl.com/ubwtq2c
25. tinyurl.com/usm6zas
26. tinyurl.com/te4e6xb
27. tinyurl.com/tmnwm4a
28. tinyurl.com/jx8oucm
29. tinyurl.com/y7czfja6
30. tinyurl.com/ruzdwuo
31. tinyurl.com/y8e6jdfx
32. tinyurl.com/y7so7jhl
33. tinyurl.com/qtol6em
34. tinyurl.com/qtol6em
35. tinyurl.com/s7jdwbx
36. tinyurl.com/sm93nzn
37. tinyurl.com/sm93nzn
38. tinyurl.com/sfqj63t
39. tinyurl.com/wsgdzob

Chapter 9 Energy and Fatigue

• ConsumerLab.com quotes are from:

1. "B Vitamin Supplements Review (B Complexes, B6, B12, Biotin, Folate, Niacin, Riboflavin & More)," Product Reviews, last updated September 1, 2020, tinyurl.com /ya3vxjvd.
2. "Nutrition Bars & Cookies Review (For Energy, Fiber, Protein, Meal Replacement, and Whole Foods)," Product Reviews, last updated

October 20, 2019, tinyurl.com /y3nsyp4h.

• *Natural Medicines*™ quotes are from:

1. "Caffeine," Professional Monograph, last updated July 24, 2020.
2. "Panax Ginseng," Professional Monograph, last reviewed August 5, 2020.

• Quote from Meredith Worthington, PhD, is from an email communication, January 14, 2020.

1. tinyurl.com/y4c4dyh6
2. tinyurl.com/slkcfwe
3. tinyurl.com/yxmbl847
4. tinyurl.com/slkcfwe
5. tinyurl.com/rr5hldw
6. tinyurl.com/yxd9e3sm
7. tinyurl.com/y3slqs4b
8. tinyurl.com/y3slqs4b
9. tinyurl.com/y5xvdv7z
10. tinyurl.com/y2yxmblx
11. tinyurl.com/y2o8jpdu
12. tinyurl.com/y5xvdv7z
13. tinyurl.com/y5xvdv7z
14. tinyurl.com/yykom73c
15. tinyurl.com/uc7em2n
16. tinyurl.com/yxdcqjc7
17. tinyurl.com/yynvrxatf
18. tinyurl.com/yxd9e3sm
19. tinyurl.com/y4tfrmea
20. tinyurl.com/yxmbl847
21. tinyurl.com/yy88afjs
22. tinyurl.com/yyggkue8
23. tinyurl.com/yxmbl847
24. tinyurl.com/y4xg6v9n
25. tinyurl.com/y6yapnn9
26. tinyurl.com/yxmbl847
27. tinyurl.com/y4g87bud
28. tinyurl.com/yyggkue8
29. tinyurl.com/yyggkue8
30. tinyurl.com/yxmbl847
31. tinyurl.com/yxhwx7q7
32. tinyurl.com/y5n738bw
33. tinyurl.com/yxd9e3sm
34. tinyurl.com/yyggkue8
35. tinyurl.com/hnhk3o5
36. tinyurl.com/y4g87bud
37. tinyurl.com/y596ojxq

38. tinyurl.com/yybtsanj
39. tinyurl.com/yxmbl847
40. tinyurl.com/yxmbl847
41. tinyurl.com/y3mzsunt
42. tinyurl.com/y6ed3xba
43. tinyurl.com/y52939n6
44. tinyurl.com/y52939n6

Chapter 10 Gastrointestinal Health—Part 1

• ConsumerLab.com quotes are from:

1. "Digestive Enzyme Supplements Review," Product Reviews, last updated May 4, 2019, tinyurl.com/uc52eda.
2. "Probiotics Review (Including Kombucha and Pet Supplements)," Product Reviews, last updated September 11, 2020, tinyurl.com/sb9x5kd.

• *Natural Medicines™* quotes are from:

1. "Align Probiotic Supplement by Align," Commercial Products.
2. "Bifidobacteria," Professional Monograph, last updated September 18, 2019.
3. "Pancreatic Enzyme Products," Professional Monograph, last updated April 28, 2020.
4. "Probiotics," Professional Monograph, last updated July 10, 2020.

• Quotes from Meredith Worthington, PhD, are from an email communication, January 14, 2020.

1. tinyurl.com/ycgws3ss
2. tinyurl.com/y6y4r568
3. tinyurl.com/slf9ufo
4. tinyurl.com/wmd3vub
5. tinyurl.com/yd33gvz7
6. tinyurl.com/y8zhjv8z
7. tinyurl.com/y8zhjv8z
8. tinyurl.com/y8zhjv8z
9. tinyurl.com/ybflykut
10. tinyurl.com/ud77rdd
11. tinyurl.com/y2qyt7lz

12. tinyurl.com/y2w37ldb
13. tinyurl.com/tny4n8m
14. tinyurl.com/yx7st8to
15. tinyurl.com/tny4n8m
16. tinyurl.com/y2qyt7lz
17. tinyurl.com/ybflykut
18. tinyurl.com/ybflykut
19. tinyurl.com/ybflykut
20. tinyurl.com/snjpxvo
21. tinyurl.com/y2gml26w

Chapter 11 Gastrointestinal Health—Part 2

• ConsumerLab.com quotes are from:

1. "Supplements for Irritable Bowel Syndrome (IBS)," ConsumerLab.com Answers, September 21, 2019, tinyurl.com/v7g3j73.
2. "Top-Rated Vitamin and Supplement Brands and Merchants for 2020 Based on Consumer Satisfaction," ConsumerLab.com, February 25, 2020, tinyurl.com/sdabzq4.

• *Natural Medicines™* quotes are from:

1. "Align Probiotic Supplement by Align," Commercial Products.
2. "Bifidobacteria," Professional Monograph, last updated September 18, 2019.
3. "Blond Psyllium," Professional Monograph, last updated August 4, 2020.
4. "Peppermint," Professional Monograph, last updated July 10, 2020.
5. "Probiotics," Professional Monograph, last updated July 10, 2020.

1. tinyurl.com/yca2hscg
2. tinyurl.com/y4spjov5
3. tinyurl.com/y4spjov5
4. tinyurl.com/y4vml7or
5. tinyurl.com/y8b6qag2
6. tinyurl.com/y8b6qag2
7. tinyurl.com/y32u6ppd
8. tinyurl.com/y8b6qag2
9. tinyurl.com/t29r5rj

10. tinyurl.com/tn6cglb
11. tinyurl.com/tcxbdwd
12. tinyurl.com/y2qyt7lz
13. tinyurl.com/y2qyt7lz

Chapter 12 Gastrointestinal Health—Part 3

• ConsumerLab.com quotes are from:

1. "Probiotics Review (Including Kombucha and Pet Supplements)," Product Reviews, last updated September 11, 2020, tinyurl.com/sb9x5kd.

• *Natural Medicines™* quotes are from:

1. "Bismuth," Professional Monograph, last updated January 17, 2020.
2. "Calcium," Professional Monograph, last updated September 1, 2020.
3. "Magnesium," Professional Monograph, last updated September 25, 2020.
4. "Probiotics," Professional Monograph, last updated July 10, 2020.

• Quotes from Meredith Worthington, PhD, are from an email communication, January 14, 2020.

1. tinyurl.com/wmd3vub
2. tinyurl.com/r3d4p24
3. tinyurl.com/unlpqd4
4. tinyurl.com/vr8hljr
5. tinyurl.com/y2qyt7lz
6. tinyurl.com/szp469k
7. tinyurl.com/szp469k
8. tinyurl.com/szp469k
9. tinyurl.com/szp469k
10. tinyurl.com/yd33gvz7
11. tinyurl.com/y2qyt7lz
12. tinyurl.com/rjo8xfh
13. tinyurl.com/ttotpu8
14. tinyurl.com/qnx7red
15. tinyurl.com/s4db3zy
16. tinyurl.com/wnsrygf
17. tinyurl.com/wfbsvmb
18. tinyurl.com/sa7pht2
19. tinyurl.com/s9c8zxb
20. tinyurl.com/uec35r3
21. tinyurl.com/rj7lvcp
22. tinyurl.com/wnsrygf
23. tinyurl.com/w7xm6ml
24. tinyurl.com/vexzv7p
25. tinyurl.com/v4srmty
26. tinyurl.com/qw24wdh; tinyurl.com/y6z3tlwr
27. tinyurl.com/w7xm6ml

Chapter 13 Healthy Hair and Hair Loss

• ConsumerLab.com quotes are from:

1. "B Vitamin Supplements Review (B Complexes, B6, B12, Biotin, Folate, Niacin, Riboflavin & More)," Product Reviews, last updated September 1, 2020, tinyurl.com/ya3vxjvd.
2. "Supplements for Hair Loss," ConsumerLab.com Answers, tinyurl.com/y2qnvom5.

• *Natural Medicines™* quotes are from:

1. "Atlantic Cedar," Professional Monograph, last updated December 16, 2019.
2. "Beta-Sitosterol," Professional Monograph, last updated March 4, 2020.
3. "Hair loss," Comparative Effectiveness Chart, last accessed October 2, 2020.
4. "Lavender," Professional Monograph, last updated September 11, 2020.
5. "Pumpkin," Professional Monograph, last updated July 24, 2020.
6. "Saw Palmetto," Professional Monograph, last updated July 20, 2020.

• Quotes from Meredith Worthington, PhD, are from an email communication, October 15, 2020.

• Quotes from Robert Griffith, MD, are from email communications, February 2020.

1. tinyurl.com/yxn7rfgd
2. tinyurl.com/qnzvlov
3. tinyurl.com/y66tbcx5
4. tinyurl.com/y68frqwj
5. tinyurl.com/ye3kg24z
6. tinyurl.com/yesm8frr
7. tinyurl.com/swmrq8f
8. tinyurl.com/yx3jclv7
9. tinyurl.com/yj7a76df

Chapter 14 Heart Health, Hypertension, and Heart Attack

• ConsumerLab.com quotes are from:

1. "Collagen and Magnesium Rise in Popularity, as Fish Oil and Curcumin Dip in Latest ConsumerLab Survey of Supplement Users," February 29, 2020, tinyurl.com/vtvdq4o.
2. "Dark Chocolates, Cocoa & Cacao Powders, Nibs, and Supplements Review—Sources of Flavanols," Product Reviews, last updated August 11, 2020, tinyurl.com/op2nvpg.
3. "Fish Oil and Omega-3 and -7 Supplements Review (Including Krill, Algae, Calamari, and Sea Buckthorn)," Product Reviews, last updated September 25, 2020, tinyurl.com/3lud98j.
4. "Top-Rated Vitamin and Supplement Brands and Merchants for 2020 Based on Consumer Satisfaction," ConsumerLab.com, February 25, 2020, tinyurl.com/sdabzq4.

• *Natural Medicines*™ quotes are from:

1. "Cocoa," Professional Monograph, last updated July 29, 2020.
2. "Fish Oil," Professional Monograph, last updated September 30, 2020.
3. "Natural Medicines in the Clinical Management of Hyperlipidemia," Clinical Management Series, November 1, 2019.
4. "Natural Medicines in the Clinical Management of Hypertension," Clinical Management Series, February 1, 2019.
1. tinyurl.com/yyffle3x
2. tinyurl.com/ltxspf9
3. tinyurl.com/sozoax6
4. tinyurl.com/ltxspf9
5. tinyurl.com/rppmteg
6. tinyurl.com/uctqfth
7. tinyurl.com/j43vz9n
8. tinyurl.com/uctqfth
9. tinyurl.com/y6y4r568
10. tinyurl.com/wqrv4m8
11. tinyurl.com/y36l3sk8
12. tinyurl.com/z3cobd6
13. tinyurl.com/wun85c8
14. tinyurl.com/sz8mc4q
15. tinyurl.com/y928bf86
16. tinyurl.com/y564gykl
17. tinyurl.com/h3wdjc7
18. tinyurl.com/nvzwylj
19. tinyurl.com/yc6lkm6k
20. tinyurl.com/y9hokww5
21. tinyurl.com/yc6lkm6k
22. tinyurl.com/y9hokww5
23. tinyurl.com/tazz9w2
24. tinyurl.com/yyp2fld8
25. tinyurl.com/yyfvqgn5
26. tinyurl.com/yyfvqgn5
27. tinyurl.com/sbkjkzq
28. tinyurl.com/qldrb7l
29. tinyurl.com/urrfyn3
30. tinyurl.com/ro2x4mv
31. tinyurl.com/ro2x4mv
32. tinyurl.com/svfqdo5
33. tinyurl.com/zxvgldg
34. tinyurl.com/ro2x4mv
35. tinyurl.com/y3mg43vz
36. tinyurl.com/ro2x4mv
37. tinyurl.com/p9pyao8
38. tinyurl.com/sxcpugv

Chapter 15 Immune Health

• ConsumerLab.com quotes are from:

1. "Airborne to Pay $30 Million for Deceptive Advertising of Cold Remedy," Recalls and Warnings, August 14, 2008, tinyurl.com/r8aqes5.

2. "Emergen-C Settles False Advertising Lawsuit," Recalls and Warnings, January 28, 2014, tinyurl.com/qtlzt6l.
3. "Vitamin D Supplements Review (Including Calcium, Vitamin K, Magnesium, and Boron)," Product Reviews, September 25, 2020, tinyurl.com/yycm7wzc.
1. tinyurl.com/wgs7cbc
2. tinyurl.com/y6y4r568
3. tinyurl.com/ydfmwoop
4. tinyurl.com/yx2t48oz
5. tinyurl.com/ua8ngdz
6. tinyurl.com/yx2t48oz
7. tinyurl.com/tnzjepm
8. tinyurl.com/sgn9s7f
9. tinyurl.com/wgs7cbc
10. tinyurl.com/tb2mlxy
11. tinyurl.com/sgn9s7f
12. tinyurl.com/wff9qo5
13. tinyurl.com/sgn9s7f
14. tinyurl.com/y6weu2on
15. tinyurl.com/tnzjepm
16. tinyurl.com/rjo67nc
17. tinyurl.com/yad6296p
18. tinyurl.com/tb2mlxy
19. tinyurl.com/ua8ngdz
20. tinyurl.com/u9bfvvn
21. tinyurl.com/wgs7cbc
22. tinyurl.com/uf4nlpw
23. tinyurl.com/so4cqg8
24. tinyurl.com/sgn9s7f
25. tinyurl.com/t62p4tf
26. tinyurl.com/ua8ngdz
27. tinyurl.com/ua8ngdz
28. tinyurl.com/wgs7cbc
29. tinyurl.com/tb2mlxy
30. tinyurl.com/wgs7cbc

Chapter 16 Keeping Skin and Nails Young

• ConsumerLab.com quotes are from:
1. "B Vitamin Supplements Review (B Complexes, B6, B12, Biotin, Folate, Niacin, Riboflavin & More)," Product Reviews, last updated September 1, 2020, tinyurl.com/ya3vxjvd.
2. "Collagen Supplements Review," Product Reviews, last updated August 14, 2020, tinyurl.com/yz8htnsz.
3. "Do Sugar Bear Hair Vitamins Really Work?," ConsumerLab.com Answers, tinyurl.com/yhc553gj.

• *Natural Medicines*™ quotes are from:
1. "Alpha Hydroxy Acids (AHAs)," Professional Monograph, last updated August 21, 2020.
2. "Biotin," Professional Monograph, last updated September 18, 2020.
3. "Collagen Peptides," Product Monograph, last updated September 11, 2020.
4. "Hyaluronic Acid," Professional Monograph, last updated February 20, 2020.
5. "Natural Medicines in the Clinical Management of Aging Skin," Clinical Management Series, December 1, 2017.
6. "Vitamin C," Professional Monograph, last updated September 18, 2020.

• Quote from Meredith Worthington, PhD, is from an email communication, December 6, 2019.

• Quotes from Robert Griffith, MD, are from email communications, February 2020.
1. tinyurl.com/y6y4r568
2. tinyurl.com/y5x6h38u
3. tinyurl.com/y5x6h38u
4. tinyurl.com/ycpdn5p8
5. tinyurl.com/yj3m59wj
6. tinyurl.com/yxwogjnj
7. tinyurl.com/y577bsoj
8. tinyurl.com/w37k97x
9. tinyurl.com/vw9dl8s
10. tinyurl.com/vw9dl8s
11. tinyurl.com/tjwgwpl
12. tinyurl.com/tjkytyj
13. tinyurl.com/ycszplkr
14. tinyurl.com/ya5l4ty5
15. tinyurl.com/uzccxas
16. tinyurl.com/qlwtzmq
17. tinyurl.com/tt75fg9

18. tinyurl.com/tt75fg9
19. tinyurl.com/u4p36nj
20. tinyurl.com/uo23ndf
21. tinyurl.com/uo23ndf
22. November 2020 issues of *Pharmacist's Letter* and *Prescriber's Letter*, tinyurl.com/yydon6qr.
23. tinyurl.com/ukjgg45
24. tinyurl.com/yawl7v4o
25. tinyurl.com/y2lfdupr
26. tinyurl.com/y5x6h38u
27. tinyurl.com/ydsmopdg
28. tinyurl.com/voezlp9
29. tinyurl.com/yhjk9b4t
30. tinyurl.com/yzummmwr
31. tinyurl.com/yhboltjk
32. tinyurl.com/yhjk9b4t
33. tinyurl.com/ttd3bbu

Chapter 17 Losing Weight

• ConsumerLab.com quotes are from:

1. "Can Psyllium Help Control Hunger and Appetite?," ConsumerLab.com Answers, tinyurl.com/vrk3jg2.
2. "CLA (Conjugated Linoleic Acid) Supplements Review (for Slimming)," Product Reviews, last updated September 2, 2015, tinyurl.com/y3s3pvla.
3. "Psyllium Fiber (Metamucil) for Decreasing Appetite," ConsumerLab.com Answers, tinyurl.com/vrk3jg2.
4. "Weight Loss Supplements Review (7-Keto DHEA, Forskolin, and Stimulant Blend Supplements)," Product Reviews, last updated May 24, 2019, tinyurl.com/y6nopo6d.

• *Natural Medicines*™ quotes are from:

1. "Alpha-Lipoic Acid," Professional Monograph, last updated August 18, 2020.
2. "Blond Psyllium," Professional Monograph, last updated August 4, 2020.
3. "Conjugated Linoleic Acid," Professional Monograph, last updated August 21, 2020.
4. "Dietary and Lifestyle Interventions for Overweight and Obesity," Clinical Management Series, December 1, 2019.
5. "Hydroxycut by Hydroxycut," Commercial Products.
6. "Natural Medicines in the Clinical Management of Hyperlipidemia," Clinical Management Series, November 1, 2019.
7. "*Phaseolus vulgaris*," Professional Monograph, last updated March 12, 2020.

• Quotes from Meredith Worthington, PhD, are from email communications, July 21, 2019, and March 22, 2020.

1. tinyurl.com/qudcl8x
2. tinyurl.com/yxul6pat
3. tinyurl.com/jkkjv95
4. tinyurl.com/jca89t4
5. tinyurl.com/u9ls6j5
6. tinyurl.com/s3d3xlz
7. tinyurl.com/yy89tbn8
8. tinyurl.com/y6tc8fjx
9. tinyurl.com/yy89tbn8
10. tinyurl.com/yxul6pat
11. tinyurl.com/y2s6fxsa
12. tinyurl.com/y54jljlw
13. tinyurl.com/y54jljlw
14. tinyurl.com/y54jljlw
15. tinyurl.com/wcbljmp
16. tinyurl.com/ydy3se9n
17. tinyurl.com/wwtxa6h
18. tinyurl.com/y4dvwrdy
19. tinyurl.com/y4dvwrdy
20. tinyurl.com/y54jljlw
21. tinyurl.com/y3wjenzc
22. tinyurl.com/s7jtglm
23. tinyurl.com/jkkjv95
24. tinyurl.com/yb5uxcnq
25. tinyurl.com/y59eedzg
26. tinyurl.com/qvbw3qd
27. tinyurl.com/t7o7cyu
28. tinyurl.com/uue7g85
29. tinyurl.com/tggulyt
30. tinyurl.com/rm5ocvl

Walt Larimore, MD, has been a family physician for forty years. The best-selling author of the Bryson City books and *The Best Medicine*, as well as dozens of other books, hundreds of articles, and nearly one thousand publications in all, he has been called "one of America's best-known family physicians" and was the recipient of a lifetime achievement award from Marquis Who's Who in 2019. He writes a bimonthly health column, "Ask Dr. Walt," for *Today's Christian Living* magazine and formerly hosted the *Ask the Family Doctor* show on Fox's Health Network. He has been a guest on a wide variety of television and radio shows, including *The Today Show*, CBS's *Morning Show*, CNN's *Anderson Cooper 360*, and several Fox News programs. Dr. Larimore currently lives in Colorado Springs, Colorado.

CONNECT with DR. WALT

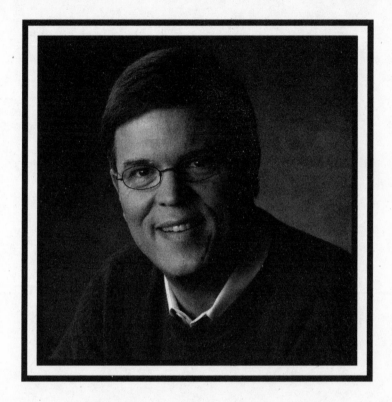

To learn more about Walt Larimore, MD, and read his blogs, visit

DRWALT.COM

We regret that Dr. Walt will not be able to answer your individual medical and pharmaceutical
questions. These should all be directed to your personal physician or pharmacist.

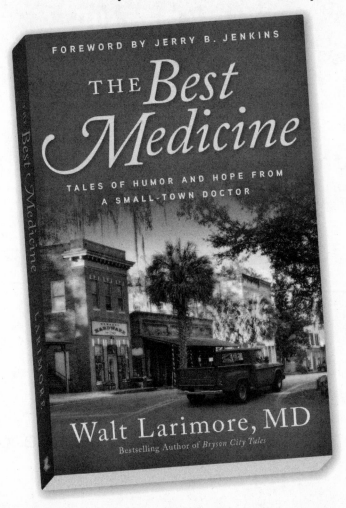

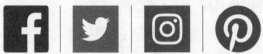
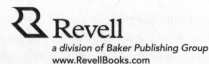